CERTIFIED FINANCIAL PLANNER™

# AMANDA HAYES-BLOCKSOM

# MEET YOUR
# BOSS

**7 STRATEGIES TO TAKE CHARGE OF YOUR
LIFE, LOVE, AND FINANCIAL FUTURE**

Published in the United States of America.
BrightRay Publishing ® 2024

*This book is dedicated to my mom, whose unspoken challenges as a woman came into clearer focus as I navigated my own path toward healing. Her journey, subtly echoing through mine, has been a guide in my quest for understanding. This work is also a homage to my inner self—the me who weathered the storms, braved obstacles, and emerged more resilient.*

*I also want to acknowledge the countless women whose paths have connected with mine. Their stories, strengths, and battles have enriched my understanding, broadened my perspective, and infused this book with a broader human experience. May the words in this book inspire every reader to face their own challenges, appreciate their inner strength, and embark on their own transformative path.*

# TABLE OF CONTENTS

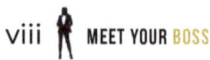

# FOREWORD

## A DIVINE CONNECTION—
## EMPOWERING THE BOSS WITHIN

In life, we often come across people who have a profound impact on our journey. Sometimes, these connections are so powerful that they feel divinely orchestrated as if the universe conspired to bring two souls together. Such is the case with my dear friend, Amanda. What began as a simple client-practitioner relationship has blossomed into a transformative bond that has left an indelible mark on my life.

As I reflect upon the time we have spent together, it is impossible to overlook the sheer strength and determination that emanates from Amanda. She is a woman who not only talks the talk but walks the walk. Her success in business is evident, but it is her emotional and spiritual growth that truly sets her apart as a remarkable individual.

Amanda has embarked on a journey of self-discovery, delving deep into the recesses of her being to uncover and release trapped emotions that once held her back. She recognized that in order to unleash her full potential, she needed to address the negative subconscious programs that had taken root within her psyche.

Through unwavering commitment and determination, she confronted these inner issues head-on, bravely peeling away the layers that obscured her true essence.

But Amanda didn't stop at releasing emotional baggage; she understood that true transformation required more than just healing wounds from the past. She diligently put into action the necessary steps to become the most successful version of herself. With unrelenting resolve, she carved out a path paved with dedication, perseverance, and unyielding faith. Through her actions, Amanda has demonstrated the power of merging personal growth with tangible goals, proving that the two are not mutually exclusive but rather intrinsically linked.

It is through our connection that I have had the privilege of witnessing Amanda's remarkable journey firsthand. In sharing her triumphs and tribulations, she has become a beacon of inspiration, igniting a fire within my own soul. Her work ethic, love, and spiritual development have served as a constant reminder that we are capable of achieving greatness when we align our passions with our purpose.

While Amanda's expertise has undoubtedly enriched my life, it is her genuine care and steadfast belief in my potential that have truly transformed my perspective. Together, we have embarked on a shared journey, a sacred pact to uplift and empower one another. The lessons learned, the insights gained, and the love shared have forged an unbreakable bond. We are united in our pursuit of personal growth, committed to nurturing the boss within and embracing the divine connection that has brought us together.

As you read through the pages of this book, may you be inspired by Amanda's remarkable story of transformation. May you recognize the power that lies within, waiting to be unleashed. May you understand that by releasing trapped emotions, conquering negative subconscious programs, and taking intentional action, you can become the most successful version of yourself.

It is my hope that Amanda's journey will ignite a flame within your heart, reminding you of your own limitless potential. May her story serve as a guiding light, encouraging you to embrace your inner girl boss and forge your own path to greatness.

Remember, dear reader, you too possess the power to make extraordinary things happen. May this book be a catalyst for your own personal and professional transformation, and may you discover the divine connections that await you on your journey to becoming the best version of yourself.

With love and endless possibilities,

Melody Robin

# INTRODUCTION

I pride myself on being put together. Even when life was overwhelming, I always made sure to "look" like I was in control. Perhaps you've felt the need to do this. The need to wear a mask of composure, even when it feels like you're moments away from a meltdown inside. Sometimes, we march on even when what we need to do most is to pause. We all navigate through a mental push and pull as our minds constantly juggle contrasting thoughts and emotions.

There are countless reasons why we may feel the need to push on, but the bottom line is it's downright detrimental to our health. We may unintentionally train ourselves to function under chronic stress. It's problematic. From heart diseases to mental health strains, not taking control of this issue can reduce the quality of our lives or, worse, shorten our time on this earth. The ironic twist? Sometimes, we're sprinting toward a goal we never truly set. By working through this book, you're not just unraveling the enigma of your life; you're unlocking a path to *aligning* your mind and body, revealing an even greater potential that's been hiding in plain sight—potential that can then be directed toward real, intentional ambitions.

This quest for reaching your innate, greater potential is what I call achieving your "Boss" status; it's the untapped power and clarity that we can embrace to

 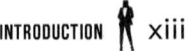

know what is genuinely right for us. It's strong, efficient, and nurturing, and it works 100 percent for you. If you're doubting its strength right now, that's okay—perhaps that's what drew you to this book. Let's be clear: it's not necessarily an inner monologue or external voice you hear; this "Boss" is the conscious awareness behind those thoughts. Some people would refer to this as your intuition or your gut feelings.

If you frequently struggle with making decisions, personally and professionally, or are tired of making the same poor decisions, then this book is for you. You don't need to run your own company or manage millions to meet your "Boss." Your age or gender doesn't matter either because a "Boss" is inside of all of us. Through these chapters, you'll learn how to trust your internal guide and quiet the sway of external voices. No matter the stage of life you're in, embracing this inner leadership is the stepping stone to taking control of your own life.

Discovering your inner Boss isn't just about setting and achieving goals; it's about a different kind of journey, one that demands introspection and a true understanding of yourself. The work of a Boss is no simple task. It requires a supportive team, the right resources, and a keen understanding of the multifaceted nature of life and human behavior.

In navigating my own life, I've shaped a strategy centered on seven essential spheres. These spheres are not just categories; they're foundational pillars that influence our well-being and the world we engage with. As you dive deeper into understanding these

 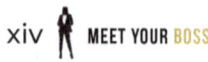

spheres, you'll recognize their significance and how they collectively form the blueprint of a balanced and fulfilling life:

- Mindset and thoughts
- Health and wellness
- Communication and relationships
- Love and emotions
- Business and finances
- Environment and lifestyle
- Faith and spirituality

Many times, we forgo strength and success in one area of life to focus on another. While there doesn't seem to be enough time in the day to fully engage in each of the seven spheres, deep commitment to each can make it feel like time has extended beyond its usual 24 hours. This is about finding a balance, not sacrificing one aspect of life for another. It's about understanding that every choice we make shapes our path and that, by the end of this book, you'll be equipped with insights and strategies to transform your life with a newfound sense of purpose and balance. With this focused growth, life won't feel as stressful or overwhelming, even when it gets busy or intense. But to reach this level of growth, you need to construct a game plan or strategy to optimize your spheres and unlock the power within you. If you don't learn how to elevate yourself and intentionally engage with the different spheres as they rotate, you will only become more vulnerable to life's stressors.

For years, I survived life's chaos through pure determination. Whether born out of obligation or desire, my intentions propelled me into territories I was ill-equipped to navigate. Guided—or, I suppose, *misled*— by the echoes of my past, setting personal boundaries became an arduous task. In my eyes, life was an ever-present race to the finish line, a race that seldom offered applause or accolades. This perpetuated an ego-driven belief that the emotional toll I was paying was simply the cost of admission, piling up and eventually hindering my growth in multiple aspects of life: my personal relationships, career, and financial stability. In my heart, I sensed there was more for me to experience, and I was tired of being held back by this invisible barrier. I needed to understand its origins, even if life didn't present me with a clear choice—until, suddenly, it did.

I remember it all came to a tipping point on the eve of my 35th birthday. Every day leading up to it, I found myself caught in a whirlwind, trying to catch whatever life hurled at me; I was operating in reactive mode, never mastering the art of saying "no." For years, I burned the candle at both ends, mistakenly equating constant stress as a badge of honor. I even joked that I might look like a show pony, but underneath, baby, I'm a racehorse. A high-functioning, stressed-out, never-pausing-before-the-next-event racehorse. Every moment felt like a stolen one; there was little room for genuine self-reflection, so all I could do was react.

I felt as though I was dedicating every waking moment to work and attempting to make my romantic

 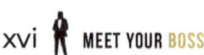

relationship perfect, though I was never truly making real progress in either one. Financially, my business was growing steadily, and to the outside world, I appeared to be the Boss of my life, exactly as I'd always envisioned. Yet, this was merely a veneer. Beneath that polished surface, a storm of doubt and self-criticism raged within me. My self-worth hinged on achievements, validation, and external praise, even if they were as tiny as breadcrumbs (and some were). The mere thought of revealing my imperfections or making mistakes held me captive. With no clear boundaries, I frequently compromised my own needs and desires in relationships. I lived under the shadow of a debilitating belief: disappointing someone was a personal failure. I mistakenly assumed the responsibility of managing other people's emotions, and in turn, I allowed behavior that was unkind, disrespectful, and disloyal. And then, one day, all of it exploded within me. It was as if I was being fired from my own dream life because I wasn't making the cut.

There I was, curled up in my bed at three in the morning, tears streaming down my face like a relentless river. Only a few weeks before, I had endured a heart-wrenching end of a significant relationship. The relationship had gotten so toxic that every day felt like a warzone. I had to walk away (literally) lest I get trapped in the throes of an Emmy-winning soap opera. I had finally reached a point of being so numb that I just didn't care. It had me questioning: was I beaten by life? This pain and drama I had allowed—was it finally enough to break me? Stress took over every aspect of my life. I was

 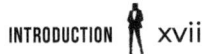

grappling with a side business (completely outside the realm of my financial practice) that had spiraled out of control. Managing employees seemed like a Herculean task, and time was a luxury I didn't possess. The cost of maintaining the operation exceeded its output—it was a financial sinkhole. Harassment was a regular ordeal at my primary work, and unhealthy coping mechanisms had become my solace. Isolation and numbness were my unwelcome confidants. It felt like there was no peace in sight, and there never would be.

Everyone wanted more from me; everyone expected me to give because I had *always* given, all done without a word of complaint. Now I felt like a weary racehorse being put out to pasture. I felt drained and empty as if I could never make anyone happy, especially myself. I was convinced that everything was my fault and that no one wanted to take any responsibility or step up. People seemed to dismiss me with ease, increasing my doubts about my self-worth. It was no longer about genuine appreciation for who I was; instead, my worth was reduced to the utility I provided or the fleeting moments of distraction I offered. The world around me appeared to be engaging in a superficial dance, treating emotions as mere games rather than heartfelt expressions. I yearned for genuine connections, for authenticity, and had grown tired of hollow charades. The weight of feeling unappreciated felt insurmountable, casting me into an abyss of pain and confusion. It felt as if I had reached rock bottom. This wasn't who I was. I wasn't the Boss of my life—I didn't even feel like Amanda anymore. I was just existing, living each day in survival mode.

 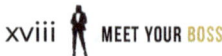

My hands were sweaty, my mind was racing, my stomach was empty, and my heart was shattered. My hands frantically sought out every accessible over-the-counter medication. Drugs had never been a part of my life, yet I was standing over Tylenol and Midol, contemplating their deadly potential. I was unsure of how to execute this ultimate act of surrender, but a lifetime of watching movies on TV suggested an overdose could be lethal. A voice inside my head, almost detached, suggested a simple solution: swallow the pills and end it all. "Time to close this chapter," it said.

I had always been a fighter, never one to shrink back from obstacles. Yet, years of accumulated trauma and a jaded perspective on life shaped my decisions in that dark moment. My fight-or-flight mode was triggered, and I felt ready to fly away toward what I imagined to be peace. I had no words to say to myself. Clutching the pills and about to make what I thought was my final decision, my eyes somehow locked onto one of those cheap tchotchkes you buy at Home Goods: a shallow earring dish inscribed with the words "Sparkle and Shine." For reasons unknown, I couldn't stop looking at it. It gave me pause, and my hand steadied. My breathing calmed, and I went to bed as if nothing had happened.

I thankfully did not go through with my intentions that night. However, it was also my turning point, the moment when I realized that I needed a major change. How did I even allow this thinking into my head? It seems so drastic, an out-of-proportion response, and yet so many people reach this point because of the constant,

 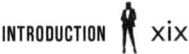

slow burn of negativity that develops over time. Then one day, it breaks in. From that moment, I saw how quickly a split-second decision can end everything. A moment of pain and sadness can take it all away forever. If you feel like this is forming in you or if you have felt these moments before, take special note. Life can be better, and you don't have to settle for less. If you feel like you've reached this low point, reach out to someone—a friend, family member, or therapist. Help is available all around you. Don't push yourself to fight this battle alone.

Remember that you are in control here. Are you ready to commit to *you*? Do you want something different? If so, now is the time to put in the work. I'm not going to pretend that my path is the "right" or "easy" one, but it's the one that turned my life around since that breaking point many years ago.

I will say that the lesson is clear: mastering your mind is the first step toward authentic freedom and fulfillment. I took that first step right after my (thankfully) failed attempt. I told myself that starting right now, I was going to commit to trying—to do the work for myself and be the Boss of my own life. I wanted all of the doors of conditioning, stress, trauma, attachment, sadness, the negative stories I was telling myself, all of it, to swing wide open. Rip the Band-Aid off and do the work. I was ready for change. The next morning, I woke up and found myself driving to a local church. Suzi, a woman I knew from town, had encouraged me to join her at church just a few months before, so I thought, *Let's do this. Let's get out of your comfort zone, Amanda.* Or, as I like to call it, your *dis*comfort zone. (Because the irony here is that we think this is comfortable, but we actually have just gotten used to discomfort and are calling it normal.)

I'd never held a deep religious conviction, but the previous night's ordeal compelled me to seek support. I needed something to lean on. I could not have even imagined the overwhelming embrace of dozens of strangers as I entered the doors. "Hi," "Good morning," "Welcome," "How are you doing?" The congregation welcomed me with open arms. Suzi was there as well, greeting me with a beaming smile and a warm hug. She was beautiful, the ultimate "show pony," except it wasn't all show. There was something very different about her. It was intoxicating, and her energy pulled me in. The pastor was a rock star, engaging the entire crowd as they held onto his every word. I could hardly stay focused, but from the depths of my own thoughts, I heard the pastor say, "Are you listening to a voice or an echo? Because an echo sounds like everything else, but a voice is clear." It got me thinking—what was I choosing to listen to? What was actually at the heart of the messages I was hearing? I needed to do some reflection here. The notion that there is too much information out there is sound. We live in a world of options, but with those choices comes confusion (echoes).

What echoes are influencing your perceptions and decisions? Here's the thing about communication: talking is only half of the equation. You need to listen, and that's difficult to do when your mind is overloaded with information and is creating doubt every second. Are you ready to listen to a clear voice of authenticity?

 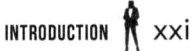

You can start by changing what you allow yourself to listen to. Monitor the thoughts you put into your mind every day.

Back in that church, I started to think: if I listened to this pastor just once a week, how would my life improve? If I listened to him two to three times a week, how would it improve? What if I started listening, reading, and consuming positivity every day? How would my mindset improve? I mean, it was worth a shot, and I had no other leads to follow. Full steam ahead, right? I knew I needed to fuel my body for power and my mind for purpose. I didn't want the short-term fix of self-improvement goals; I wanted this to be a complete evolution of myself, a commitment to long-term change.

As Tony Robbins believes, people attract what they put out.[1] Attraction is a reflection of our own energies. If we are enmeshed in negativity, how can we hope to draw positivity into our lives? The inability to attract and sustain the positive was a mirror to my internal world. This realization sparked a burst of determination. I needed to:

- Take control of my mind and reprogram my thinking;
- Fuel and strengthen my body;
- Understand my insecurities;
- Distill my finances and business;
- Own my now; and,
- Become my own Boss!

If you are setting out to meet these same goals, the methodology and tips in this book can serve as a basic guide for comprehensive transformation. The work isn't easy, but each approach is meant to be utterly accessible so you can successfully implement it. This book seeks to open up and normalize conversations about the struggles associated with finding your self-worth and net worth. While these topics can often feel intimidating or isolating, they don't have to be. With the right approach, understanding, and strategy, you can master these domains, breaking free from the endless cycle of self-doubt and analysis paralysis. Through my experiences in the world of finance and the lessons I've learned in life and love, I hope to illustrate that the foundational principles of each sphere are intertwined so that you can rise to the top in each one.

As you read further, consider your "risk tolerance." This is often used in reference to finances, but it does have a broader application. Risk tolerance is about how much uncertainty we can manage without feeling overwhelmed. On the other hand, "risk capacity" focuses on the necessary risks required to meet our aspirations. Basically, there are risks we're *willing* to take and those we *must* take in order to achieve our goals. Occasionally, a gap forms between what we're comfortable with and what we need, creating a challenging balance to strike. I want to encourage people to stop making excuses, stop being their own worst critics, and stop using their insecurities as an excuse for bad behavior. Growth is uncomfortable, but you have to embrace this discomfort

 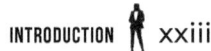

to make next-level progress. Let my experiences serve as examples and my strategies help steer you toward a life rich in purpose, fulfillment, and true joy. The most important move is the one you make next!

# 01

# Rising from the Echoes: Assessing the Journey to Self-Evolution

I wasn't always so emotionally aware. I grew up in what I would describe as a peaceful bubble, blissfully ignorant of what adults were doing or discussing most of the time. From what I can remember, my childhood was pleasant, well-protected, and conditioned by the idyllic world my parents had created for my brother and me. We learned about life primarily through our parents' actions and teachings. While I didn't grow up wealthy, I knew the importance of money and the hard work required to earn it. My dad, a staunch advocate for hard work, played a significant role in shaping this mindset. His perspective on the world was strict and influenced by his complex feelings toward success. He fought relentlessly for something he simultaneously seemed to resent. Unknowingly, through his actions, he instilled in me the notion that validation and attention were paramount, often at any price.

As I stepped into adolescence, the tranquility of our childhood cocoon began to show cracks. The sobering facets of adulthood started to ripple through my consciousness, and I couldn't help but notice the subtle shifts in our family dynamics. The peaceful bubble of my early years started to fill with the never-ending noise of my parents' loud arguments. No matter where I was in the house, I could hear their angry voices echoing off the walls. It felt as though I was a spectator in an ongoing, domestic bout where no championship was at stake—only the erosion of my parents' happiness. My father's voice became a palpable force of dissatisfaction while my mother's confidence seemed to wilt under the weight of it all. What struck me the most was that this

 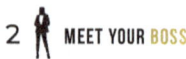

animosity had been masked so well before, hidden from us like an unspoken secret.

As I unintentionally tuned into their dialogues, a simple question would often occupy my thoughts: *Why can't they just get along?* I imagined, like many kids my age, that I could fix things between them (or so I thought). The issues had become so intense that they just didn't care about their surroundings or the repercussions.

Have you ever been in a situation like this, one where you can't control your emotions? My parents struggled within their relationship for years before reaching this boiling point. Raised without the benefit of positive role models themselves, they became increasingly consumed by the challenges of their own relationship and began to progressively neglect my brother and me. While I couldn't articulate it at the time, their growing emotional distance profoundly affected both of us. As I transitioned out of high school and started to take control of my own life, I chose to pursue a degree in psychology in college. My aim? To assist people in understanding themselves and improving their interpersonal relationships— especially my parents.

## FROM PSYCHOLOGY TO FINANCE

My venture into psychology was propelled by a profound curiosity I had developed from these echoes of my family atmosphere and a desire to assess and understand the complexities of human behavior. I had this grandiose vision that studying psychology would provide me with perfect clarity and secret insights into every aspect of existence. Who needs a crystal ball when you have a psychology textbook! My freedom to explore these questions also allowed me to explore the world. I was no longer in my parent's bubble—I was ready to *GO*.

Still unaware of how my upbringing had pre-programmed me, I continued to grow up with quite a rebellious spirit, which guided my actions and led me to make impulsive decisions. At the age of 18, I found myself engaged to be married, yet stuck—I didn't want to get married, but my partner had convinced me that I wouldn't find anyone better. A solid selling point, right? Given the emotional chaos at home, I had no one to turn to for advice. I didn't know how to trust my gut, so I listened to my partner's voice. It was a nonsensical argument, yet somehow, it held sway over me for months until my tiny inner boss, a flash of intuition, yelled, "STOP! *What am I actually doing?*" She was faint but potent enough for me to call off the engagement before any wedding plans could be solidified.

Throughout college, I got caught up in promotional events that took me all over the country. It was like I had a stake in Delta Airlines. I was balancing school and work and moving in all directions, seemingly driven by an unknown force in me. I pushed boundaries at every turn, and I continued to let my environment influence my actions more than I should have. These adventurous and chaotic experiences thankfully served as invaluable lessons along the way. I was like a detective on the hunt for the ultimate truth, armed with nothing

 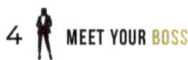

more than a notebook, a credit card, and curiosity. However, I faced an insurmountable obstacle: not everyone wanted help nor were they open to change, regardless of my enthusiasm to assist.

It became clear that many people were more interested in filling their internal voids with superficial distractions—be they shallow relationships or material possessions—rather than confronting their issues head-on. They seemed content listening to echoes instead of making concrete changes to their unfulfilling habits. I had to face the reality that people give away a lot of free time for pleasure hunts while ignoring true values. When the pleasure fades, they move on and seek out more. The field of psychology was not as black and white as I'd hoped, and I craved a solution handbook that was more straightforward and more definitive. It just wasn't working for me.

Long story short, I changed majors. Acting on the advice of a guidance counselor, I ventured into the world of marketing—and it felt like a breath of fresh air. The dynamic environment, catchy taglines, and vibrant community seemed as though they had been custom-designed for me. It turns out that sometimes veering off-course can lead you directly to a path that's a much better fit.

# THE BOYS' CLUB

My "aha" moment arrived during an international marketing class in my junior year of college. Everything started to align perfectly. A representative from Edward Jones, a highly regarded investment firm, visited our class to discuss "finance as a career path," and he instantly caught my attention. The crisp, gray suit, smart shoes, and commanding presence said, "I'm put-together." *This* was what a man looked like; this guy was in charge. More than anything, I wanted to have that kind of presence—for people to listen when I spoke and respect what I had to say.

As he spoke about the finance world, I found myself strangely intrigued. Finance seemed so straightforward, so black and white. I mean, what could be more crystal clear than math? It was like a tantalizing puzzle just waiting to be solved. My professor, a tiny blonde pistol of a woman, saw my interest and encouraged me to pursue an opportunity with Edward Jones. I wasn't used to this kind of encouragement, having been told for years that a college degree for me would be nothing more than a "sheepskin on the wall." I wasn't sure I could tackle this. Yet, I couldn't shake the thought of it. My interest was sparked, and the challenge was created. I was going to go for it, no matter what anyone said, even when my dad told me just before my first interview, "You'll never make it in finance; it's a boys' club."

*What on earth was a boys' club?* And why was he suddenly saying this to me? My whole childhood, I was never told I couldn't do something just because I was a girl. In fact, I stood out for it. I wanted to do everything my older brother did because I thought he was the coolest. I played baseball, basketball, volleyball—you name it, I wanted to try it. When my dad suggested that finance was some exclusive boys' club, it rubbed me the wrong way. Scratch that, it didn't just rub me the wrong way; it set my determination on fire! I had to fight for this just like he taught me. I never let being a girl stand in my way before, and I sure wasn't about to start now. I didn't need fancy labels like "bad b*tch" or "girl boss." Nope, I just wanted to be a BOSS, plain and simple. And my one and only speed was *GO!* It couldn't be that hard. Could it? I dove in.

Driven by curiosity and a desire to be a part of this so-called "boys' club," I took the most enticing opportunity that presented itself fresh out of college: a position at Edward Jones. I wasn't going to assess my worth based on others' judgments. I was ready to pursue the goals others had frequently dismissed. It was time for me to take charge of my life, be self-reliant, and discover what new skills this journey would demand of me. Could this be the first day of my dream job? I was prepared to find out.

The firm hired me almost instantly. It was a pivotal, historical moment when women were boldly making strides in traditionally male-dominated fields and truly excelling. Pioneers like Ruth Bader Ginsburg and Maggie Walker had already paved the way for young women like me. My entrance into the finance industry sparked not only professional achievements but also a wave of personal growth. Today, as the founder and president of Aurion Wealth and Aurion Wealth Advisors, I am living a life far beyond what that little girl decades before could have ever envisioned. It's an astounding testament to how far curiosity and determination can take you. So, let's look at some revealing facts on where women in business stand now. Let their success inspire you to take a leap, challenge yourself, overcome adversity, and infiltrate the "boys' clubs" in every business.

- Forty-two percent of all businesses in the U.S. are women-owned.

- Women-led businesses employ 9.4 million workers and generate $1.9 trillion in revenues annually.

- States with the most women-owned firms are Hawaii, Virginia, and Colorado.

- More than 1,800 new women-owned businesses are created each day in the U.S.

- One in three female entrepreneurs has experienced sexism as a business owner. *(UGH, seriously?)*

- The top priority of women-owned businesses is to get more funding and financial help.

- The average loan size for women-owned firms is 50 percent *lower* than for male-owned.

- Thirty-one percent of female business owners have school-aged children at home.[2] *(How's that for needing to choose between a career and family?)*

Even if you're the only woman with a seat at the conference table, the number of women in business is on an upward trajectory. Here they are: women who are not just organizing events but challenging norms, shattering ceilings, and paving a significant path for numerous women around the globe. True success is rarely achieved without overcoming barriers—any obstacles we may face in the battle just prove how big of an impact we are going to make when we come out on top. Maintain unwavering faith in the mission you've undertaken. Believe in the cosmic rhythm—the universe has a unique way of orchestrating triumphs for those of us who fight strong. This moment, however challenging, will soon become a cornerstone of resilience and growth in your narrative. Wear that as a badge of honor, ladies!

## RECOGNIZING THE INVISIBLE CHAINS: A NEW FOCUS

Within each of us resides a unique energy that resonates in response to our surroundings and experiences. This resonance manifests as either positive or negative vibrational frequencies, which, in turn, shape our emotional state. While some of these "symptoms" or emotional signatures can be positive, those arising from negative or traumatic experiences tend to create destructive cycles of emotions like depression, addiction, anger, or withdrawal. Such negative cycles become self-reinforcing because they feed our innate need for safety or control. It's a classic case of starving the soul to feed the ego or excessively avoiding past sources of pain and thereby losing our present and future. These behaviors are limiting and drag us away from reaching our full potential.

It's a habit we have to consciously break by unlearning the behavior that may have served us through the worst of times but is out of place once we are safe. An example would be a neglected child seeing attention as essential as water. They would love a glass of clean water, but they will drink dirty water to survive. They may act out and create situations to get attention no matter how self-destructive it appears. Receiving that attention reinforces that negative behavior. Again, it doesn't matter how "bad" for them it is down the road— it's about the instant payoff. To escape this loop, we need to consciously unlearn harmful behaviors.

I wasn't immune to this self-destructive cycle. Emotional gaps in my life made me susceptible to unhealthy early relationships. I mistakenly equated that dirty water with clean water, just like I described above. Dodging an ill-advised marriage at 18 should have been an alarm bell, but I found myself entrapped in another similar situation just as my finance career was about to take off. Entangled with a man who was far older and incredibly deceitful, I was thrown into a whirlwind of lies so complex that it threatened my newfound career path. This manipulation silenced the assertive inner voice I once had as a young adult. At that stage in my life, I lacked the tools to untangle myself from such deceit.

Thankfully, my dad stepped in before the situation deteriorated further. However, his critical and condescending approach made me withdraw from ever confiding in him again. I learned that attention wasn't synonymous with love. My insecurity drew me into the relationship, but it was my ego that kept me there, craving an apology and proof of change that never came. I thought I needed this validation, not realizing it was just more dirty water. Instead of seeking clean water, I assumed this was the norm. It took me a while to realize I couldn't control others, only how I responded to them.

We all learn at different speeds; it's critical to recognize the importance of emotional self-reliance. Start developing a supportive network that will hold you accountable to do better each day. Ask yourself, "What kind of water am I drinking?" You may not have fancy Fiji water, but it should at least be clear.

As I entered my new career with Edward Jones, I had no room for distractions. Being rebellious was exhausting, and it pushed me into too many situations that my core personality and beliefs were not suited for. I turned inward, mistaking isolation for focus. My propensity for "going full throttle" shifted from seeking attention in relationships to being absorbed in work—a trap commonly known as being a workaholic.

## VEGAS, BABY

My early workaholic tendencies made me buckle down and commit to the finance industry—I was going to succeed; there was no alternative. I can only imagine the difficulties women faced in all the years before me. Breaking into certain industries means overcoming stereotypes and proving yourself to be just as valuable as "one of the guys." It's the unfortunate reality of being a woman in the professional world. One of my earliest professional experiences with the boys' club cliché was when I visited Las Vegas for an investment conference. I was seven years into my career, and the year was 2013. Out of the 600 advisors in attendance, only 10 were women, hence the "boys' club." During the event, I was like a magnet for men trying to charm me with their questionable flirting skills, trivializing my finance career like it was a pretty pink purse. Some even invited me for drinks, blatantly showing off their wedding rings as if they were of no concern. I already had a negative perception of men prior to this trip due to failed personal relationships, but to experience that behavior in the professional world was disheartening. Where was that sharp, kind, intelligent man I'd met in my marketing class?

I was left wondering if I needed to get a degree in eye-rolling or just accept this behavior as "the norm" to succeed in my profession as well. But it wasn't just the men—the women were also harsh critics. Most were intensely competitive and conniving. It was a challenge to figure out who to trust and keep in my circle. It left me questioning if I would even have a circle of friends or a partner I could trust. People would say, "Eh, that's just business; don't take it personally," but I did. I took it *all* personally.

But then, a light-bulb moment: what if personal and professional spheres weren't so separate after all? Could it be that people's behavior in business settings is merely an extension of their personal disposition? This breakthrough made me realize that strategies for improving my personal life could also be applied in a professional context. After all, if business had nothing to do with personal interactions, human resources wouldn't be investing in training videos about "appropriate workplace conduct."

For a long time, I had been laboring under the belief that I could only count on being let down by people, and this cynicism led me to construct a metaphorical "wall of protection" around myself. While this shield seemed necessary, it had the unintended consequence of pushing away genuinely good people. I began to question the very foundation of my previous relationships. Was I sabotaging them with this invisible barrier? Was *I* the common denominator? Was I the one who needed to change rather than make changes around me?

Change is seldom easy, even when beneficial. Often, we gravitate toward people who validate our complacency rather than those who challenge us to grow. Hiding behind my self-erected wall was easier than facing the difficult work of self-improvement. But as time went on, the composition of my inner circle evolved. While some remained steadfast companions, riding life's turbulent waves alongside me, others disembarked along the way. Each person, however, left an indelible mark—be it as a valued friend or a cautionary tale, everyone contributed to my ongoing journey of self-discovery and growth.

## CONFUCIOUS IN MY PHONE

One of my closest friends, Ramey, is more or less a lifelong pen pal, going strong for over two decades. Though he resides on the other side of the country, we first crossed paths at a comedy show in St. Louis during an Edward Jones new advisor training trip—a serendipitous meeting that forged a friendship for the ages. Over the years, I've poured my heart out to him about all sorts of relationship woes and personal challenges—every issue imaginable. He's been a steadfast source of support, a rock through thick and thin. But in our nearly two-decade friendship, he's raised his voice at me exactly twice. Let me share the first instance with you.

As much as we'd like it to, growth doesn't happen overnight. I'd found myself in a few other unhealthy relationships, faced yet again with disrespect and betrayal. This time, Ramey had had enough of my echoes. Instead of being the usual sympathetic ear, he erupted in anger over the phone. "Listen," he said, his voice tinged with a fury I'd never heard from him before. "Wake up. This is on you! You're the one tolerating these behaviors. These people are all the same; they all follow the same patterns as toxic fools! You're choosing this life, and you don't even want it." His words landed like a sledgehammer, echoing in my mind for days afterward.

What he said was a bitter pill to swallow, but he was absolutely right—I was constantly grumbling about the same old problems yet never lifting a finger to change anything. I was allowing people to feel comfortable hurting or disrespecting me. That dirty water was like an IV being pumped into my veins for survival. Ramey's the kind of friend you need in your support system: someone who isn't afraid to dish out a hearty serving of tough love when you need it most. Sometimes, it's precisely that sort of raw, no-holds-barred honesty that propels us into action. Ensure that the principle of "tough love" is reciprocated though. Avoid getting consumed with a friend who frequently offers criticism but refuses to accept any in return. I've ended several relationships in my life due to this hypocrisy.

If you're reading this book, you must know and accept that it's time to make some changes. Awaken your curiosity, and start by looking for the common denominators in your past situations. Why do you get stuck in the same situations and patterns? It's easy to play the victim, but growth comes when you square your shoulders and take responsibility for your role in these cycles. For me, it was clear that navigating these complexities would require a thoughtful game plan— one that was straightforward, uncomplicated, and consistent yet adaptable to my evolving understanding of myself. Challenges inevitably arose, and my desire to heal forced me to shift my perspective from victimhood to a learning mindset. Instead of asking, "Why is this happening to me?" I began to ask, "What can I learn from this experience?" But this realization was only the beginning. The patterns are invisible to most of us because that's how we get through life. We build the walls through our experiences, and we conveniently hide behind them when we feel afraid or challenged. This is a pointless feat that will stunt your growth. Luckily, at some point, I realized each of us is responsible for the life we lead. You can leave a toxic relationship, whether it's a friend or a lover, but if you don't heal what attracted you to that person, you will just meet them again. Same drama, different person. The wounds might not be your fault. But the healing *is* your responsibility.

I can't write one book and automatically fix every reader's problems. This book doesn't encompass every known experience, as some of us have had truly unimaginable traumas that need far deeper advice and support than what this book offers. We are all dealt different cards in life. Some of us start on first base, some of us look like we are permanently in home-run land, and some of us are hardly in the dugout. Everyone is going to have a different starting point, path, and outcome.

One time, I found myself thinking that a change in location and experience would be the solution to my problems. Well, guess what? Negative behaviors are not constrained by geography. I have witnessed numerous people fall prey to tactics such as intimidation, guilt, and manipulation, regardless of where they live or travel. You have to start asking yourself if these are truly coincidences of meeting "the wrong person" or "choosing the wrong investment," or if they are patterns where the root cause can only be changed by looking inside yourself. Learning how to listen to that inner Boss voice, and make it a real Boss, is key. We can either make excuses, or we can make decisions. Prepare yourself to become a one-person force of nature, unstoppable in the pursuit of authenticity.

# 02

# The 7-28 Method

My mom would always tell me, "If you want it, Amanda Kim, I know you will find a way to get it." If someone told me no, I heard, "Yes." I always saw a "no" as an opportunity to go and find a way. As I shared earlier, my dad's authoritative nature and high expectations for my brother and me shaped much of my early life. Looking back, I believe his intentions were rooted in wanting us to succeed, to surpass our expectations. It was like he had a secret mission to turn us into superheroes or something. In his unique manner, he wanted to give us the kind of nurturing and positive affirmation he never got from his father.

While he did teach us passion, grit, and determination the best he could, he also passed down the torch of less positive traits like people-pleasing, materialism (specifically Money Worship, which we'll get into later), and emotional detachment. To gain his approval, I tirelessly practiced to excel in all kinds of sports, which he enjoyed as he was usually the team coach. He demanded greatness, but just as his father held back, my dad was never very affectionate. I can't recall ever getting praise unless I did something *exceptional*. And even then, it was a very lax reward system. Excellence was the default, the expectation, and I did not want to disappoint. If you're not careful, you can spend the rest of your life trying to fulfill the demands of others without pausing to consider your own wants and needs. We're constantly surrounded by people—family, friends, or coworkers—and their expectations for us.

I came to realize many years later that we need to get approval from ourselves, first and foremost. Otherwise, we're just putting on a show of living, and for what, societal approval? Unrealistic expectations? Your life, love, and financial future are at the mercy of your mindset. It is *your* life; shouldn't *you* have the final say? Shouldn't *you* be in charge? It's easy to answer "yes," but it requires an intentional effort on our part to think and act as if *we are* the Boss of our lives.

## REALITY CHECK

I need you to stop and ask yourself: what does a snapshot of your life look like today? If you're having trouble assessing your life right now, consider the questions below. You might not like the answers, but you have to accept what's going on right now. This exercise isn't limited to your career or relationships—it's a holistic reflection, spanning emotional well-being to finances. It's designed for anyone, regardless of life stage or occupation, and I use it as a personal assessment.

- Do you feel stuck with how to get from where you are now to where you want to be?
- Are there challenges that keep resurfacing on your quest? If so, what are they?
- Are you unsure about how to effectivley manage your life, love, or finances?
- Are you ready to shift your mindset and habits to achieve a more fulfilling life?

For years, my behavior and patterns engineered the negative situations and consequences that weighed me down. I reached a breaking point. No longer could I let my ego and insecurities duke it out nor could I entertain the voice that kept whispering, "You can't do this." It was time to listen to that other, softer voice that was saying, "Yes, you can." We all have choices, and I had been making the wrong ones. My endless rationalizations built a towering skyscraper of excuses: the wrong partner, career, business decisions—you name it.

If this resonates with you, you're likely nodding your head. It's comforting to blame external circumstances, isn't it? But here's the twist: the real obstacle is you. This doesn't mean you're a failure; it means you need a reset. Your habitual actions perpetuate your current reality. In essence, you've been recycling the same old, dirty water and pretending it's thoroughly hydrating.

"My idea of a group decision is to look in the mirror."
— Warren Buffet[3]

So, are you ready for a change? Ready to lead a balanced life that includes happiness, love, and financial stability? Follow me as I introduce you to the method that helped me break free: the 7-28 Method.

## THE SPHERES OF YOUR LIFE

The 7-28 Method essentially works as a diagnostic tool to pinpoint challenges in your life and provide solutions for how to address them. I believe your life can be divided into seven core areas. This book encapsulates all that I have learned through my journey—it's a personal narrative rather than a scientifically grounded theory or complex manual. It revolves around the seven spheres, which I mentioned in the introduction, and they function as "checkpoints" to guide you when you feel lost. Reflecting on the questions below will help kick-start your journey toward self-improvement.

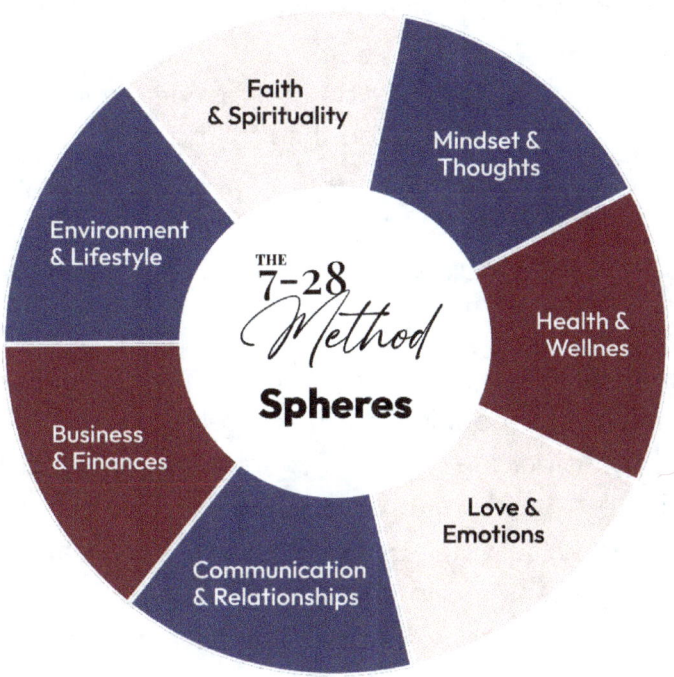

**Mindset and thoughts:** This sphere focuses on your mental approach to life's challenges and opportunities. It examines your resilience, your capacity for growth, and the general tone of your thought patterns.

- How do you respond to adversity and challenges in life?
- Do you possess a growth mindset that encourages learning from experiences?
- Can you identify the predominant tone of your thoughts? Is it positive, negative, or neutral?

**Health and wellness:** This sphere is concerned with your physical well-being and lifestyle choices. It looks at your engagement in physical activities and your strategies for coping with stress.

- How does your daily lifestyle reflect your commitment to your health and wellness?
- Do you engage in regular physical activity that you enjoy?
- How do you actively manage and mitigate stress in your life?

**Communication and relationships:** This sphere deals with your interpersonal skills and relationships. It asks you to consider the quality of your interactions and your ability to set and maintain boundaries.

- How do you nurture and sustain meaningful relationships in your life?
- How do you feel after most conversations—energized or drained?

- Are you comfortable and skilled in setting and maintaining healthy boundaries?

**Love and emotions:** This sphere explores your emotional intelligence and how emotions play a role in your decision-making. It also dives into your understanding and practice of love in various relationships.

- Do you allow your emotions to guide your decisions, or do you feel controlled by them?
- Can you distinguish and cultivate healthy love, not just in romantic relationships but in all aspects of your life?
- How much priority do you give to nurturing your emotional well-being?

**Business and finances:** This sphere looks at your professional life and financial health. It encourages you to consider if your career aligns with your core values and whether your financial decisions are balanced for the short, intermediate, and long terms.

- Does your career align with your core values and provide a sense of purpose?
- Do you make business and financial decisions based on long-term goals or immediate needs?
- Are you confident in your financial literacy and capability to manage your finances?

**Environment and lifestyle:** This sphere focuses on the physical spaces you occupy, such as your home and workspace. It looks at whether these environments are conducive to your well-being and productivity.

- Do the environments you inhabit, including your home and workspace, reflect and support your aspirations and well-being?
- Does your home environment offer comfort, tranquility, and inspiration?
- How does your workspace contribute to your productivity and creativity?

**Faith and spirituality:** This sphere explores the role of spirituality or faith in your life. It considers how these beliefs offer comfort and how they influence your interactions with others.

- How does your faith or spirituality provide comfort, strength, and guidance in your life?
- Is your connection with your faith or spiritual beliefs nourishing and satisfying?
- How does your spirituality or faith practice influence the energy you project onto others and the world around you?

Your answers to these questions can shed light on which areas of your life need a little more attention and show where to focus your efforts. The seven spheres function like your personal board of directors: interconnected and influential over each other.

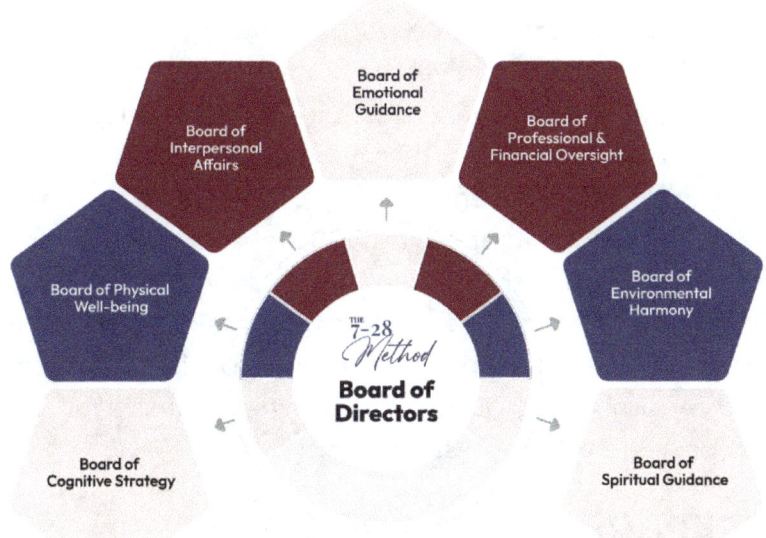

Each of these "boards" can offer guidance, strategies, and best practices for managing the corresponding areas. As the chairman and CEO of your life, it is your responsibility to cultivate harmonious relationships with all members of this board as they are your essential life spheres. The "7" in the 7-28 Method embodies these seven spheres, seven board members, and seven days in a week—a testament to the unwavering, daily commitment needed for self-improvement and growth. As the Boss of your life, you are accountable for everything that happens in your existence. And this requires a 24/7 commitment.

The "28" in the 7-28 Method symbolizes an aspirational expansion of time: when you get your life together, you often feel like you've been granted extra hours in the day, as if you have 28 instead of the usual 24. This number is also inspired by my birthday, July 28, which is fittingly in the seventh month of the year. (Yes, I'm a Leo!) Before I ever crafted my 7/28 Method, I used to look at the clock when the needles pointed to 7:28 and affirm to myself, "I'm amazing, and I'm doing wonderfully." It was my initial attempt at fostering a positive mindset and reframing my outlook, even when I wasn't feeling my best—to this day, I still do this!

## PREPARE FOR PROGRESS

Healing isn't linear. It's unique to each individual, paced by their rhythms of recovery. Getting through my parents' divorce was no different; it was a clumsy dance of stumbles and course corrections. I was sent to therapy, but as a defiant teen, I clung to an uncompromising stance: "This is who I am. Love it or leave it." It's only now that I realize how self-destructive that mindset was and how it magnetized all the wrong kinds of attention my way. You start playing in the Toxic Band, and there's no shortage of people willing to encourage that negativity. I kept this perspective for years and through a series of therapists. It wasn't until more recently that I changed my tune. I had a series of wake-up calls and began to build my arsenal of strategies to strengthen my mind and attitude. Then, at that pivotal moment in my bathroom at 3 a.m. when my entire life seemed to come to a tipping point, I knew I couldn't keep it up any longer. Something had to change; I needed to make real progress. This desperate need prompted me to solidify the 7-28 Method as a way to transform my life and improve my seven spheres, one day at a time.

The key to healing is consistency and dedication. It won't happen overnight, and sometimes, you may lose a battle with yourself. Just grit your teeth and prepare to win the war. Good leaders never give up. I tell myself that I am the general, not the soldier. You may take one step forward and two steps back, and that's okay. Most people focus on the result, not understanding the path to get there and what that takes. I know my journey has included missteps and some backward moves (which I like to call failing-forward steps) followed by determined strides up the mountain. My own life isn't some magical fairytale of an emotionally intelligent and savvy woman starting her own firm. I had a series of positions at firms that didn't appreciate my skills and a few exes who were a long way from Prince Charming. We can't allow these situations to define us. It's easy to point at external forces like the economy, your ex from high school, your parents, or even the car that cut you off in the Chick-fil-A line! People who choose to complain about these things will likely stay complainers until they have a wake-up moment. Instead, choose to move forward.

The life I have today—one of professional success and personal evolvement—came about because I learned from my experiences. I learned to ask for more from others and, more importantly, myself. I learned to communicate my needs and develop myself instead of justifying toxic behaviors. Above all, I learned that success in all areas takes consistency.

Don't worry if you're feeling a bit lost in your personal or professional journey; it's perfectly normal. Recognize this is a huge step forward, even if you're not quite sure of the solution yet. The important thing is to decide that *this* is the moment to get back on track and recalibrate your thinking. Begin with adjusting your mindset and integrating new habits that align with the life you desire. Use these habits to break free from the procrastination trap of "I'll start tomorrow." It's time to put away the excuses and embrace the challenge. Get ready to set your targets and dive into action; your journey of growth and evolution is about to start! The understanding you seek is just around the corner, and every step you take brings you closer to it. Keep reading, keep learning, and keep moving forward.

## HOW TO A.C.H.I.E.V.E.

I'm not about to pretend that making life changes is as easy as reading, learning, and moving forward. You have to take the work step by step. Upon recognizing your seven spheres and reflecting on your responses to the proposed questions, you may identify certain areas that demand immediate attention, or you may find that every sphere could use some refinement. That's perfectly alright. The A.C.H.I.E.V.E. approach provides seven strategies that you can begin to employ within each sphere. This equips your "board of directors" with a detailed blueprint to enrich every facet of your life.

1. **Assess the situation**
   - **Take a reality snapshot:** Look at your current life, relationships, and financial status through an unfiltered lens.
   - **Identify gaps:** Spot the areas where you're not meeting your goals or expectations.
   - **Embrace honesty:** Be brutally honest with yourself; denial won't lead to improvement.

2. **Curiosity**
   - **Question patterns:** Investigate whether you're stuck in recurring cycles or patterns in various aspects of your life.
   - **Seek signs:** Notice any coincidences or signs that might offer insight into your situation.
   - **Challenge assumptions:** Don't accept things at face value; dig deeper to understand the "why" behind your current state.

3. **How and who**
   - **Identify resources:** Determine what skills, people, and tools you need to move forward.
   - **Build a team:** Actively seek out mentors, colleagues, or partners who can help you achieve your goals.
   - **Skill up:** Invest in yourself by learning new skills or enhancing existing ones to meet your objectives.

4. **Initiate proactive steps**
   - **Create an action plan:** Develop a concrete, step-by-step plan to reach your goals.
   - **Prioritize:** Focus on the most impactful actions that will bring you closer to your objectives.
   - **Start now:** Don't wait for the perfect moment; take action today.

5. **Execute with precision**
   - **Follow through:** Ensure that each action you take aligns with your plan.
   - **Pay attention to detail:** Don't gloss over the small things; they often make the biggest difference.
   - **Adjust as needed:** Be prepared to pivot your approach based on feedback and results.

6. **Visualize success**
   - **Envision mental imagery:** Create vivid, detailed mental pictures of the success you aim to achieve.
   - **Form emotional connections:** Attach positive emotions to these images to amplify their motivational power.
   - **Practice regularly:** Make visualization a consistent part of your daily routine.

7. **Evaluate progress**
   - **Set milestones:** Break your goals into smaller, measurable milestones to track your journey.

- **Have regular check-ins:** Periodically assess your progress to ensure you're on the right path.

- **Celebrate wins:** Acknowledge and celebrate even the small victories to keep your motivation high.

The method is versatile enough to adapt to various circumstances. Perhaps you're the writing kind of learner. You can dedicate a journal to this self-assessment and revisit it as often as necessary. If you need additional support, this book also offers a companion workbook on our site at www.728Method.com. You can work through that at your own pace, taking these concepts further and applying them to your life. Additionally, my team and I are committed to updating and sharing new information daily via our social channels. You can A.C.H.I.E.V.E. anything you set your mind to if you're willing to work for it.

## TAKING ACTION

As we move further into this transformation together, you'll find the book brimming with deeper insights, personal anecdotes, practical examples, and useful tips that I have gathered and applied along my own path. We'll use my seven strategies not only to improve each sphere but to interconnect them, providing a comprehensive roadmap toward enduring success. This is not just about change; it's about the growth and enrichment of your entire life journey. Just like art is never finished, your life should always be a work in progress. If you settle for "good enough," it'll become a slippery slope for other toxic behaviors. That's been my experience.

As the creator of the 7-28 Method, you may have the misconception that I fully embrace its teachings every day. But no, I'm human just like everyone else. And like everyone else, I struggle and drift off course at times. That was the case at the start of 2023. I was in the middle of making huge changes in my firm. Then, surprise, I found out I was pregnant. My husband and I were delighted. Being 40 and having focused the last two decades on my career, pregnancy wasn't something I ever thought would happen for me.

Yet, joy turned to heartbreak when I miscarried at the end of the first trimester. This loss sent me spiraling. I put on more weight than I ever had before, grappled with low self-esteem, and lacked the drive to engage with my business or socialize. All seven of my spheres were impacted. The emotional upheaval from these unexpected life events was overwhelming.

However, a jolt back to reality came when a cherished early client of mine, Bob, passed away. It underscored the unpredictability of life and the urgency of fully embracing each moment. Realizing I was veering off my desired path, I revisited the tools of the 7-28 Method. I fully embraced my A.C.H.I.E.V.E strategy, implementing it rigorously across various aspects of my life. Assessing my various spheres was crucial as were proactive steps and daily actions aligned with my goals. Whether it was consistent workouts, a disciplined diet, substantial time dedicated to business innovation, or ensuring adequate rest, I put myself through a self-imposed boot camp to actualize my objectives. In just four months, I was back on track, down almost 35 pounds, and successfully launching business changes within my firms. I felt like a Boss, like Amanda, again!

# What's Holding You Back: Dismantling Barriers and Facing Fears

Navigating friendships can be as complicated as managing romantic relationships. Often, we aren't formally taught how to cultivate healthy friendships; instead, our early friendships form based on convenience—proximity to our homes or classmates in school. As we grow older, our friendships start to evolve based on our changing environments. As the saying goes, "you are the average of the five people you spend the most time with," so choose wisely.

## FRIEND OR FOE

I mistakenly believed that having stories or drama was a prerequisite for people to listen and pay attention to me. This belief stemmed from lessons I learned in childhood and an ever-growing mountain of insecurities I stacked over the years. In return for sharing these stories, I found myself surrounded by "friends" who were always eager to hear me vent. They were like emotional spectators, keen on watching the drama unfold but critical, condescending, or just plain absent when I genuinely needed help or support. For example, I had a group of girlfriends who seemed supportive but subtly undermined me with passive-aggressive comments like, "Oh, is that what you plan on wearing?" I also heard, "Sure, it's fine if that's what you think is best," and "Why do you want to work so much when you could go to the beach?" Such remarks were nothing but veiled judgments, sowing seeds of self-doubt and questioning my life choices. The odd thing was, I felt strangely drawn to this environment as if I had to drink from this "dirty well" of relationships just to quench my social thirst.

The familiarity of this type of treatment, based on my childhood, kept me from seeing the toxicity. Toxic, self-destructive behavior often feels more comfortable than healthy, self-affirming situations and relationships, and so we seek it out. The problem is the power these relationships have in our present. However, there can be no growth without discomfort. The power of your closest relationships can't be understated as you start to mirror the traits of the five closest people around you. Realizing the detrimental influence these people had on me was only the first step. I was still in the early stages of learning how to set personal boundaries, when to give my emotional energy, and when to withhold it. And I learned that in most situations when I felt "comfortable," I wasn't growing.

One of the best investments you can make is investing in yourself. As I climbed the ladder of professional success and could afford a therapist and a life coach, I realized I no longer needed to rely on this audience of "friends" for emotional validation. The moment I started keeping my struggles to myself and setting boundaries around what I chose to share, these friends began to drift away, evidently upset that they could no longer use my stories as fodder for their entertainment. When you raise your standards and take action, you may lose these types of friends from your circle, but they don't have your best interests at heart anyway. They're not yet ready to meet their Boss, but you can't let that stall you. Ditch those people; fire those people! Never forget that you are the Boss of you, and nothing can hold you back more from your true potential than toxic friends, employees, or partners. You are not responsible for other people's emotions or their shortcomings in resolving them. You become firsthand proof of what change can look like, and that scares people. When you put crabs in a bucket and one tries to climb out, the others will pull them back down. "Misery loves company" is a saying for a reason. So, make sure the people in your life are pushing you up, not holding you down.

Not long before I started writing this book, my friend Ramey and I had our second major disagreement, and it was for the same reason as before: I faced the recurring issue of allowing toxic people to be around me, whether for business or pleasure. This lesson was difficult for me to learn, and life kept sending me the invoice—payable in mental energy, financial resources, and even physical health—until I truly grasped the concept. You can't always go around things; sometimes, you have to go through them until you figure it out. But just after that second fallout phone call, I received an unexpected piece of wisdom in my mailbox. It was a postcard featuring a simple drawing of a stick figure ascending a staircase. On the flip side, a quote by Ebonee Davis was etched: "Don't be afraid of the solitude that comes with raising your standards."[4] This was Ramey's way of telling me that it was okay to elevate my expectations, even if it meant walking alone for a while.

So, now, consider me your modern-day pen pal. Though I'm not using traditional postage, I still aim to share valuable insights with you. Leave behind the fear of rejection and the dread of being alone; as Ebonee Davis realized, personal growth often comes with a measure of solitude—and trust me, the rewards are worth the sacrifice.

## FACE YOUR FEARS

It's time to explore some other obstacles that could be holding you back. Let's talk about three core fears:

1. **The fear of judgment:** People will always have opinions about what you should or shouldn't do. The key is not to let their judgments cloud your vision.

2. **The fear of haters or critics:** Some people will actively undermine your achievements. Learn to separate constructive criticism from mere negativity.

3. **The fear of making a mistake:** Mistakes are unavoidable. They're also the stepping stones to success. Own them, learn from them, and move forward.

We've all encountered these fears at some point, and if you're reading this, it's likely they're influencing your life right now. Rather than becoming mere bystanders to these fears, we can set ourselves apart by how we respond to them. Fears left unchecked can spawn excuses and misconceptions, hindering us from seizing control. Traits such as a need for attention, a disruptive nature, and a disdain for authority can be the elements that fuel these fears, but by channeling these traits positively, we can gain a better handle on our fears and keep them in check. By embracing the unknown, daring to explore new horizons, and aligning ourselves with inspiring people, we can face and master the fears that might be holding us back.

Success might imply confidence, but it certainly does not equal it. I have met many successful individuals who deeply struggle with their relationships. Let me introduce you to a client of mine named Mary. Mary juggled numerous six-figure projects for her business and had three divorces under her belt. Despite her extraordinary success, she failed to recognize her value. Instead of delegating tasks, she wore every hat imaginable—owner, maintenance, accounting, services, and follow-up. These blurred lines and her intense self-reliance left her burnt out, unfulfilled, and complacent like a stressed-out racehorse sacrificing her health for her wealth. She convinced herself she loved her job and loved her husband, but retirement and alone time couldn't come fast enough.

Mary contemplated other alternatives, but she was embarrassed to ask anybody for help due to the high regard others had for her. She prized this external image of success and was reluctant to jeopardize it. It's not a weakness to ask for help—that's how you become the Boss of your life. The mindset of "I can handle it myself," or "Everything is fine," often acts as a hurdle that prevents many people from truly owning their lives, loves, and finances. You might have heard someone say, "It's simpler just to do it myself or to be alone." This fear-driven thinking restrains individuals from instigating positive transformations in their lives. It's as if they believe no one else is capable of handling tasks, and yet they are often the most self-critical people as well.

I find those same weaknesses are quite often partnered with the strengths of resilience, endurance, grit, and fight because these kinds of people chase their goals like it's the only thing they're able to accomplish in this world. Chasing goals with fervor can be a double-edged sword. While it may get you the success you desire, it can also leave you constantly asking, "What's next?" So, take the time to give yourself that well-deserved pat on the back. Otherwise, you may find yourself running like I did, forever chasing something you don't really want.

## MEETING THE EXCEPTION

People often don't change their situation until it becomes a must-fix. Even then, it may be difficult to find the motivation. Remember, just because something isn't exciting doesn't mean it isn't worthwhile. Most good changes require consistency, which is often a struggle. Mary, the client I mentioned, still wears all the hats, though she could delegate. It takes time to make effective changes. Most float through life on the "maybe-fix" autopilot until something or someone comes along that is the exception. Maybe this "exception" is another business owner, a new relationship, or the risk of losing an existing relationship or business. Something tells them or shows them how or why to change and essentially "gives them permission" to ask for more of themselves and others. One of my "exceptions" was my ex's mother, Sherry.

Sherry was my superhero in Chanel. I was completely spellbound. She radiated brains, poise, and professionalism like Wonder Woman at a board meeting. Her outfits were as flawless as her Excel spreadsheets, and her words were strung together with the grace and precision of a master violinist. She was a B-O-S-S in the financial services industry. She was another elite show pony/workhorse like Suzi. Bottom line: Sherry commanded the room and held the respect of those around her. She fiercely defended her beliefs and her family at all costs. She was unapologetic in a way that was inspiring, and she was exactly who I needed at the time in my life. Sherry was the female version of that well-dressed man I met back in my college marketing class. The way she held herself showed me how much I wanted to change. I thought, *This woman is in control!* She took me in and mentored me like the fairy godmother of my career dreams. Being around her felt like having a front-row seat at New York Fashion Week and taking an MBA course all at once.

I longed for nurturing and supportive qualities from my mother but eventually realized that the negative traits I learned as a child were not intentional on my mother's part. She loved me and my brother and never intended to cause us harm. In reality, she had her own trauma and emotional wounds. With the limited resources available to her, my mother did the best she could to raise us. Without realizing her actions until much later, she taught me to remain quiet in response to hurtful behavior, thereby modeling the allowance of hurtful relationships for me. However, my mother lacked the accountability to acknowledge her actions as she never had a parent teach her how to do it. In contrast, I had now found a woman who taught me a different way, which I found appealing.

It was then that I began to flourish. I had this role model teaching me how to navigate the finance world as a mini-Wonder Woman, and therapists were stepping in like helpful neighbors while I unpacked my past. They took out box after box and explained what was inside.

Remember, healthy individuals have to be capable of acknowledging their shortcomings to grow and evolve positively. I'd held onto a grudge with my mother and finally had the chance to let that go. Clocking in more hours with my therapist than my favorite TV shows, I was eventually able to cut my mom some slack and serve a generous portion of forgiveness. It's been over 10 years since Suzi and Sherry, the dynamic duo, stepped into my life and created waves that still influence me today. Now, I'm ecstatic to report that my mom and I are not just in a good place, but we're like two peas in a pod.

## LEAN INTO CHANGE

It's okay if you're finally recognizing that you too have been drifting through life for years, downplaying your needs, drinking dirty water, and allowing others to be comfortable dismissing you. It's just not okay to *keep* allowing it. I told myself that I didn't mind the trade-offs for a long time—they felt familiar. For me, it took a trip to couples therapy with an ex before I realized I had been shortchanging myself. In therapy, the very place I least expected it, I found out I wanted more and, shockingly, how to get it! You know the saying about people coming into your life for a reason, season, or lifetime? Well, when this season came calling, I didn't just answer the door; I threw it open and invited it in for tea!

I unpacked more in therapy than I ever thought possible. These therapists loved psychology like I loved finance, and they were good at it. I found it fascinating to explore how the trauma of my exes and workplace drama stretched all the way back to my relationship with my parents. All of it made so much sense. How had I been floating through life not knowing this emotional code? I was hands-down a people pleaser with a Money Worship money script ingrained from my childhood. If you ever meet a workaholic or a people pleaser—or you're able to admit to being one—you can trace that quality back to parents or some pivotal parent-like relationship. This is because people pleasers begin as parent pleasers—they play the role of a cheerleader, therapist, or peacekeeper to one or both of their parents. They're used to thinking, "As long as they're okay, I'm okay," and this not only represses their voice but creates a form of emotional monitoring. It also can make you vulnerable to gaslighting because you just want everyone to be okay. The roles of parent and child become blurred, and you're forced to grow up fast. That was my story, and it took therapy for me to fully realize the impact this environment had on me.

This book has an avalanche of ideas and strategies. But remember, if you don't spring into action and implement those ideas, all this just turns into a very elaborate doodle. So, let's do more than lean in; let's do a full belly-flop into this! There are three distinctive roles people play in their interactions with others as introduced to me by my previous therapist:

- Adult-to-adult,
- Parent-to-child, and
- Child-to-parent.

This was first spelled out in the 1960s book *I'm OK–You're OK* by Thomas A. Harris.[5] The notion is so simple, but I was oblivious to it for a long time. Initially, I often found myself in child-to-parent dynamics, but over time, the roles would pivot to parent-to-child dynamics. Here's the twist though: recognizing these role-swapping performances requires an incredible degree of self-awareness! There is a tendency for our minds to misinterpret initial situations, convincing us of a reality that might not exist. As I mentioned earlier, my parents had a tumultuous divorce in which neither was emotionally present for years. My brother and I were forced to grow up fast in order to keep things in line. This carried on into my adulthood. It's no surprise that I constantly felt a sense of unease as if something crucial was missing from my life or that there was more yet to be discovered. I often found myself grappling with this unexplainable feeling of being "stuck."

The moment of clarity hit when I recognized and owned the dysfunctional family dynamic I grew up in. This realization was challenging because it felt as though I was betraying my parents by recognizing this, which made me feel very guilty and ashamed, especially since my dad was constantly telling us about all the "sacrifices" he made for our family. He then reinforced this by saying we were ungrateful any time something didn't go his way. It's tempting to see things in black and white, thinking that acknowledging dysfunction implies our parents were negative influences or that our childhoods were devoid of good moments. However, life and relationships are more nuanced—positive and negative experiences *can* coexist. While my parents did have negative qualities, they also had loads of positive traits that shaped me into the woman I am today. I can't be mad at the bad without being grateful for the good. Recognizing these unhealthy dynamics allowed me to break generational cycles, to grieve for the parents I wished I had, and to truly understand and accept them for who they are today. This forms the foundation of authentic love. It's important to heal from our past to prevent continuing these patterns and mislabeling them as "normal."

When you read about my experiences or insights, I don't want you to passively nod your head and move to the next page but, instead, consciously reflect on how these situations resonate for you. How can you put these arrows in your quiver? Can you turn it into something that's personalized to what you need in life right now?

This is why you have to decide for yourself whether you're listening to an echo—some repeated, hollow piece of advice that won't suit you—or a distinct voice. Many times, we know what we need to do but ignore the voice, saying it's "too hard" or "too much work." There can be many burdens and traumas holding you back from making the necessary adjustments to your life. It can be really hard; I get it. As one therapist, Ed King, said to me, "I can't heal a burn if you're standing in the flames." Essentially, he meant that until I'm no longer in the same mindset or situation, it's nearly impossible to make improvements. I needed to detangle myself from the situation to have the space and perspective to do the work.

The initial step toward change should be to concentrate on resolving the problems that you can actually fix. Admittedly, I tend to tackle too many issues simultaneously, which can be daunting. Attempting to correct *everything* that's "wrong" in your life can be overwhelming. Take the necessary time to make well-informed, calculated decisions and transitions. You don't have to hit all your goals at once; instead, identify the ones most important to you and work toward them first. Similar to individuals tackling debt, start by identifying the issue with the greatest impact or "interest rate." The sooner you can alleviate the more substantial burden, the quicker you'll be able to manage the remaining issues.

If you allow issues and conflicts to accumulate, you're more likely to react impulsively or lash out. Your finances are no different; overwhelming debt can push individuals into bankruptcy or to take desperate measures. While such reactive changes might occasionally bring about positive outcomes, urgent, fire-alarm changes may not always be in your best interest. I used to let my dissatisfaction in situations escalate until it became an unbearable must-fix. Driven by frustration, I'd hastily jump into the next situation without tackling the important ones first. My friend, Ramey, would often joke, "Are you alright? I assume you've already gotten a new car and changed your hair color, haven't you?"

His joke was spot-on! I ended up relinquishing so much because I failed to tackle issues before they spiraled out of control. It's somewhat like washing dishes. Doing them daily might be as fun as watching paint dry, but if you neglect them, you'll soon be greeted by an overflowing sink and a mountain of dishes that demand far more time and effort to handle. Problems can rapidly spiral out of control, and addressing them early can be a game-changer.

How about we take a moment to reflect on what you just read with a few questions:

- Are you battling wildfires while happily roasting marshmallows in the flames?
- What's that mythical boundary you've etched for yourself?
- Just how long are you planning to have this bonfire party?
- Or have you simply decided to tan in the glowing warmth?

Sketch out a list if you need to. You know nothing says "I'm in control" like a dazzling T-chart. Even a fire station operates on the ABCs of putting out fires—you also need to construct a plan!

Don't you just look at those merry, can-do folks and think, "Gosh, I wish I had that glow!" Well, the secret's out: happiness is a choice! You can't simply sit back and wait for positivity to drop into your lap. You've got to be the intrepid explorer, sniffing out the resources to support your happiness and then using your muscles to actively build it up. That's your roadmap to staying accountable and marching steadily toward progress.

# CHAPTER
# 04
# Initiating Your Roadmap

People often comment on my dedication to my business. This sphere is extremely important to me, so perhaps that's why it catches people's attention. They see my success and start to view me as if I possess some magical prowess, extraordinary capabilities, or a unique skill they lack. As much as I love words of affirmation—my top love language—let me tell you a secret: there's nothing superhuman or even special about me. I'm just a regular, hardworking woman with the same 24 hours in a day that everyone else gets. But I do have an ace up my sleeve that many people endlessly strive to find: passion. That passion pulls me to create consistency in my mind and body that gives me those "four extra hours" in the day, seven days a week (a.k.a. the 7-28 Method).

Every day, we wake up to opportunities. It's what you do with those opportunities that defines your life. Most people say, "One day, I'll do this." You and I both know that it's easy to push things off until the next day. We tell ourselves that it's okay because life gets in the way. Though we're all guilty of it, we also have to acknowledge how procrastination limits our growth and success. Life is a professional curveball pitcher, and it's up to us to step up to the plate and swing for the fences—rather than opting for the instant gratification that procrastination seductively whispers in our ears. Instead of persisting with the mantra of "one day," let's consider reorchestrating it to say, "Today is Day One." Can you discern the distinction? The former serves as a permit for delay while the other is a call to action. It's not easy, but we have to become our own personal cheerleaders to succeed here.

# BUILDING THE PILLARS: CONFIDENCE, SUPPORT, AND STRESS MANAGEMENT

I hope you're bursting with readiness to master these new skills and nurture an optimistic self-dialogue. The aim is to say goodbye to the nagging inner critic and welcome your inner cheerleader. I'm fully aware that this transition may not be seamless for everyone. You might encounter hiccups at the outset or find the breadth of the impending changes daunting and anxiety-inducing. Rest assured, this is perfectly normal. To combat this, it's essential to have a set of fundamental coping mechanisms at your disposal, ready to be deployed whenever those three familiar fears (judgment, criticism, and making a mistake) threaten to make a comeback.

## Master Stress with Box Breathing

Picture this: your heart is thumping, your palms are sweaty, your thoughts are racing—does this sound familiar, perhaps from the introduction (or even your personal experiences)? This is a typical reaction to seeing a mountain lion on your hike or, more fittingly today, spotting an ominous email from your boss with the subject line: "We need to talk." Before you hit the panic button, let's talk about box breathing—your secret weapon against stress!

We take a staggering average of 23,040 breaths daily, but how many of those are we truly aware of, especially when our anxiety ramps up? The box-breathing technique is your golden ticket to regain your calm. It is a technique often used by Navy SEALs to handle high-stress situations. Clinical studies have shown that it's effective in reducing stress hormone levels.[6] Here's how you can try it:

1. Breathe in deeply for a count of four.

2. Hold for another four counts.

3. Exhale for a count of four.

4. Wait for another four before taking the next breath.

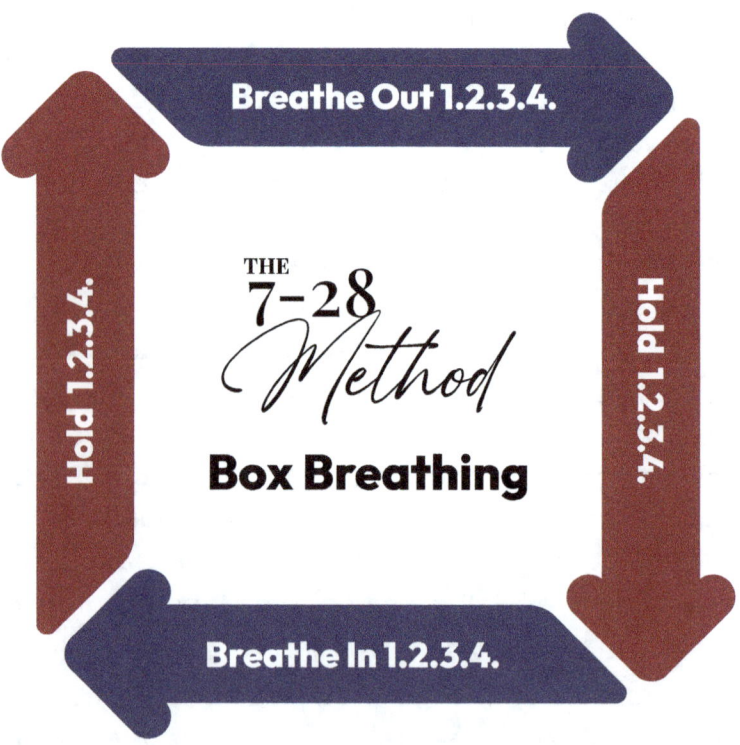

Imagine yourself drawing a box with each phase, hence the name. This method isn't just about getting more oxygen; it's a systematic reset for your stress mechanism. A few rounds of this and your body's internal dialogue will become, "No mountain lion; we're good here." Now, why is the approach so powerful? Inhaling and exhaling properly is like giving your body a free, all-access pass to a health club. It enhances energy, mitigates stress, fortifies the immune system, improves sleep quality, and accelerates recovery. With enough oxygen, every system in your body steps up its game. Who knew that the secret to becoming a Boss in life was hidden in every breath we take? So, next time you find yourself facing a stressful situation, take a deep breath and channel your inner Zen master; it's as natural as, well, breathing!

## Self-Reflection and Lessons from the Past: A Dual Compass

Every morning, I wake up grateful for my family and home, not to mention my fulfilling career. But gratitude doesn't make me complacent. Each day provides an opportunity to be introspective—to reflect on the way I interact with the world and affect those around me. This isn't about vanity; it's about responsible leadership. Like a general, I strive to embody the change I advocate, hoping to inspire others and stand out as someone's "exception."

But self-awareness isn't only about the present. It involves an understanding of your past—the triumphs, failures, and life-altering experiences that shape you. Your past is not a space you should dwell in, but it is a resource you can draw upon to navigate life's complexities. When you experience a surge of dread or anxiety, take it as a cautionary alert. Pause and assess the situation. Could you be veering toward repeating a past mistake? If so, let your history guide you toward making a better choice this time around. Use it as a reference, not as a direction to revisit.

Despite ongoing personal growth, there will always be unexpected challenges. When life threw a curveball my way—a heartbreaking loss—it could have derailed my journey of self-discovery. But instead of spiraling, I used it as a wake-up call to affirm my resilience. I now know that I'm not just a survivor; I'm a navigator, continually adjusting my course based on past and present insights. So, as you go through life, keep your eyes on the road ahead, but don't neglect the wisdom that your metaphorical rearview mirror can provide. Together, they form your dual compass—a powerful tool to guide you through the maze of life's choices and challenges.

## Harness Your Peak Hours, Build the Right Network, and LEAP!

Understanding your productive rhythm is the first key to unlocking a more efficient you. Some of us are morning birds, revved up and ready to go as soon as the alarm rings, while others come alive under the moonlight. Personally, my mornings begin at 6 a.m. with coffee and Squawk Box setting the tone for the day. On the flip side, my friend Lisa is a night owl who hits her productivity stride around 2 a.m. The point is that we both get things done during our peak hours. So, forget societal norms and find your unique rhythm to tackle your tasks effectively.

Beyond recognizing your productive time, you also need to set realistic yet challenging goals. My own task list used to be ridiculously tiny and repetitive, just so I could pat myself on the back for completing something. It was like celebrating a tiny victory every time I crossed off "breathe" or "put on pants." But with habits and routines, that list grew larger and more ambitious.

Next, consider the people in your life who potentially comprise your support network. Are they contributing to your stress or helping you navigate through it? Will they alleviate your stress or add to it? Surround yourself with people who will demand the best from you. Many people build themselves a team that automatically agrees with and validates damaging behavior. It puts you in a constant state of "discomfort," yet we tell ourselves it's our "comfort" zone. What's comfortable about being stressed or unhealthy? Continuing to adapt to this discomfort will limit your growth, and it doesn't do you any favors. You have to find new people who will support your efforts to change and encourage you to be the best version of yourself.

There is a great book by Dan Sullivan called *Who Not How: The Formula to Achieve Bigger Goals Through Accelerating Teamwork*.[7] It's the foundation of my mindset for goals: I don't ask myself *how* I'm going to get all this done anymore. I ask *who* is going to get these things done. Successful leaders surround themselves with the right people, and teamwork is how things get done. Elevating others lets you anchor your mind in abundance, not scarcity.

I once advised a client, Chris, who was struggling with a social circle that didn't serve his new entrepreneurial goals. I suggested he expand his social horizons to include mentors and other uplifting individuals. This small change can have a profound impact on your trajectory, aligning you with those who bring out the best in you. This advice may sound simple, but it follows the principle of Occam's razor: when faced with a problem, the simplest solution is often the best one. You don't need to make grandiose changes to avoid financial pitfalls or other life challenges. Sometimes, the smallest lifestyle adjustments can yield the most significant results.

Lastly, don't let self-doubt and fear stand in the way of taking bold steps. I remember that in the early days of my career, I was caught in a cycle of self-doubt, constantly convincing myself that I lacked the adequacy and sufficient knowledge to take any leaps. At the inception of my career, I found it daunting to consult a client who had $100,000 to invest, a sum I certainly didn't possess 18 years ago. The whisper of imposter syndrome sat on my shoulder, casting doubt on my competence to give sound advice. However, it's amazing what time and a slew of experiences can do. As my career started hitting its stride, it brought along some new trusty companions: bolstered confidence, enriched knowledge, and an expanded comfort zone. Now I'm at a stage where I am unshakeable, thanks to my comprehensive education and confidence. By doing the work, I have become cognizant of the value I bring to the table and possess the confidence to seize opportunities. Yes, even when dealing with clients boasting a net worth of more than $100 million.

## Walk and B*tch: Fueling the Roadmap with Wellness and Real Talk

The "game" of life isn't about perfection; it's about action. No one is born a world-class athlete; they all started with a toddler wobble. The wellness part of your sphere involves moving your body! I've fluctuated with weight gains and losses dozens of times in my life. I've been an athlete since I was a child, but I was never really aware of what to eat to be a top-performing athlete. Food is fuel, but sadly, many of us attach other meanings to it. My trainer was the first to illuminate the idea of viewing food as fuel rather than a source of comfort or even punishment.

In my younger years, I was immersed in dance, focusing primarily on ballet and jazz. A piercing memory from my past is when, at the age of 15, my ballet teacher candidly told me, "You're lucky you're pretty because you'll never be a dancer—you're too fat." This led to a two-year struggle with bulimia until a dentist's visit alerted me to the impending loss of my teeth if I continued this self-destructive behavior. Wanting to keep this from my family, I somehow managed to stop. Regrettably, I also gave up ballet class. It still bothers me to know that I didn't stand up for myself that day and, worse, that I allowed those comments to push me down instead of making me rise to the challenge. I know this happens to many people, so it's crucial to use other people's criticism as a source of inspiration rather than letting it cut you down. Instead of having those reverberate in your mind, drown them out with your own voice, reminding you to believe in yourself!

Everyone you see now who is "winning" was likely "face-planting" at some point in their lives. I had to get real with myself. I had to be honest about the excuses I was making before I could truly transform. My list was long and included everything: being tired, having to focus on my career, not having enough time to meal prep or watch calories, not knowing where to start, and not having enough support. One by one, I acknowledged my excuses. Once I became aware of them, I choreographed solutions for them. I needed accountability, so I hired a trainer to meet with daily. I know that's not a solution for us all, so how do you make room for self-improvement while life keeps throwing you curveballs?

Let me offer you a straightforward concept to ignite your fitness fire: the "Walk and B*tch" method. It's my ultimate go-to solution for venting while staying fit. My girlfriend Eva was the inspiration behind it. I was going through a tough time and didn't want to go out and face the world. She told me, "Even when life sucks, staying in bed won't change anything." The rule of this game is straightforward yet effective; if you feel the urge to complain about life's woes, do so while on a walk. Imagine venting for two hours—this means you're also walking for two hours. You'll finish feeling lighter, emotionally and physically. Odds are, your legs will run out of stamina before you run out of things to b*tch about, which might encourage you to equate being tired with being tired of venting.

However, two friendly tips: select your confidante wisely, and don't assemble a whole parade; keep the group small. No one likes a constant complainer, not even your besties. And remember, therapists are great listeners too—they're just a phone call away! Years ago, I had a bad habit of complaining about my partner. I had an army of sympathizers ready to rev me up too. I rarely spoke to friends about the good stuff and only shared when I was frustrated. I think we all are guilty of getting a little too heated after an argument with a partner. It was no surprise then that my friends weren't supportive of my relationship; they only heard me talk about it in a negative light. How you represent yourself and your life is important—you have to protect that. Otherwise, you may find yourself vilifying others and making yourself look foolish.

"Walk and B*itch" is a great tool to pull the reins on how you communicate with your intimate circle of people. A lot of the time, people don't pay much attention to how they communicate with the people they're close to, but that's just as important as a conversation with a high-level client, even if they are in two completely different spheres. If complaining is your default mode when you talk to your friends, it can significantly change their perception of you, and not in a good way. I'm not saying you can't ever complain, but keep a distinction between what you should say to a friend versus your therapist (or even just your pet).

## Hold Yourself Accountable

You need to have accountability when it comes to reaching your goals. I'm the type of person who gets easily distracted by shiny side tasks if I don't have some serious accountability parameters. It's like trying to resist the temptation of a freshly baked chocolate chip cookie. Impossible, right? I need some structure to keep me in line and focused on my goals.

Without goals, you'll wander, and when you wander, you get lost. Life is too short to spend wandering in a nebulous cloud instead of strategically working toward your goals. You have to figure out the way to get your compass back on track. You have everything it takes to achieve the same mental and physical transformation that I have. It's all about that simple willingness to give it a shot. So, when you read this book or hear my story, don't think, "Wow, she's amazing. I could never do that." No, scratch that negative self-talk. Instead, tell yourself, "If she can do it, then I can absolutely do it too!" It's time to kick those doubts to the curb and start working toward your goals like a Boss. So, is it going to be one day, someday, or is *today* going to be your Day One? Let's do this!

# 05

# Organizing Your Life Like a Boss

So far, we have explored the importance of assessing situations, getting curious, and taking account of your support system. But all that wisdom begs a big question: how do you act on it? If you're a seasoned entrepreneur, a stay-at-home parent, or someone trying to manage all aspects of life, this chapter is for you. Because let's face it: your life, your nine-to-five, and even your romantic life needs some serious organization.

## PRIORITIZE LIKE A PRO: THE DEA STRATEGY

When juggling the aspects of life, love, and financial matters, start by establishing your DEA board—your personal Discomfort Enforcement Administration! Your initial step should be confronting and controlling discomfort. I will say it again: your age, gender, or stage of life doesn't matter. You don't need to run a company or manage millions to meet your inner Boss. Everyone can benefit from a little life organization. You must learn strategies for how to delegate, eliminate, and automate.

1. **Delegate:** Identify tasks that can be effectively delegated to others. For example, you can hire a virtual assistant (or an in-person assistant) to manage administrative duties, such as scheduling appointments and organizing emails. You can set up InstaCart to manage grocery shopping or assign it to a family member. By delegating these tasks to someone else, you free up valuable time to focus on your highest priorities.

2. **Automate:** Look for tasks that can be automated using technology. For instance, if you spend a significant amount of time manually inputting data into spreadsheets, consider using software or tools that can automate this process. Hire a bookkeeper, set up online bill pay, or sign up for Zelle for more seamless processing of your expenses. This not only saves time but can reduce the risk of errors while improving efficiency.

3. **Eliminate:** Evaluate your to-do task list and pinpoint tasks that are unnecessary or low value. These tasks may consume your time without significantly contributing to your goals. Eliminate or minimize them whenever possible. For example, if attending certain meetings proves to be unproductive, consider opting out or finding alternative ways to stay informed.

This simple DEA strategy will make your available time expand before your eyes—and it's usable for everything from professional tasks to mundane chores like scrubbing your kitchen or battling the jungle that is your backyard. Ever seen the latest Shark electric vacuum? At this point, I'm half convinced it can not only sweep, vacuum, and mop but also cook a five-course dinner. (Nobody can hold a candle to my husband's cooking though—he's the best!)

Since you can't be everywhere at once, it's crucial to focus your energies on activities where you add the most value. For business owners specifically, this could mean striving to "replace" yourself in daily operations by delegating out, so you can concentrate on strategy and growth. I don't mean stop work entirely, but instead, focus on tasks that align with your highest and best use. Explore systems and processes that can reduce stressors in your business and life. Remember, no single person will solve all your issues, but adopting a new process can pay tenfold. Building a scalable, profitable, and organized business is challenging. Many entrepreneurs learn this the hard way, like my client Mary who would not ask for help. They attempt to wear every hat, and the business ends up controlling them instead of the other way around. To get it all done—the grunt work, strategic thinking, and execution—you have to start with organization and consistency.

Perhaps you're questioning your abilities, complete with a deep dive into your self-doubt. It's important to follow that up by reflecting on whether that's a realistic assessment of yourself or just your insecurities hosting a loud karaoke night. Pump up your confidence like an enthusiastic cheerleader—don't shy away from the work! If you perceive unhappiness as your "penalty" for not being enough, consider how your unresolved issues may be holding you back and think about seeking professional help. Thinking that an opportunity will only happen if it's meant to be places a lot of responsibility onto Fate's plate, and she's busy with other work!

## WHEN BUSINESS BACKFIRES: THE COST OF VENTURING OFF THE PATH

About a decade into my career, I was asked by a friend to make a significant investment into a startup business outside of my core expertise. Remember that side business I alluded to in the introduction that was stressing me out? Well, here's the back story to that whirlwind.

My enthusiasm to broaden my business horizons, coupled with my inability at the time to establish boundaries or properly underwrite alternative investments, led me to take on the challenge. As a result, I found myself in a precarious financial situation. Initially, the process appeared straightforward: devise a concept, secure a location, acquire equipment, recruit a team, and promote it all. But running a business is not simple, especially when you're already committed elsewhere. My attention was divided, and I delegated tasks to a team that I hadn't adequately evaluated for their ability to manage responsibilities, largely because I wasn't entirely familiar with the tasks myself. As the business grew, the choices became less clear, forcing me to rely more on my intuition.

Accounting became a mess. Invoices from multiple sources accumulated, challenging my efforts to discern what was valid. I was out of my depth in this new field, and it showed. My main business was doing well, but I was draining funds from it to sustain the failing side venture—a textbook example of throwing good money after bad.

Guided by my heart and my head, my intuition became a compass prompting me to dig deeper into the chaos. My findings showed that I had been overcharged in multiple sectors. The employees were engaging in dishonest practices, pitting themselves against one another in juvenile banter. I'd had products stolen, and the facilities were being abused left and right. The problems had compounded to a *must-fix*. It was the kind of experience you'd expect to see in a dramatic soap opera—a storyline filled with twists and turns that left me reeling. I had allowed this drama in, and it was time for it to leave. I sought out additional opinions, hoping that the facts would read differently. It took multiple confirmations before the harsh reality sank in—the world isn't always fair, and not everyone has your best interests at heart.

The only positive here is that I used the experience to gain a deeper understanding of human behavior, finance, and business operations. My intuition told me that there was still more to the story, and my instincts were right. I was ultimately able to address the root cause of all the business's troubles, although this came at a great price, personally and professionally. After thoroughly evaluating the side business, I found no justification for shifting my focus away from my core operations, which offered higher profit margins and resale value. I sold the side business and refocused my efforts on my core work and vision.

# CHAOS TO CONTROL: YOUR BUSINESS ROADMAP TO RECOVERY

With newfound clarity and renewed focus, I took steps to rectify the situation and put my business back on a path toward profitability. This necessitated a clear approach. Here are additional strategies that I used to guide that transformation:

1. **Assume leadership:** Show up and step up to actively participate as a leader, diving deep into all aspects of your business operations. Understanding the minutiae can empower your strategic decision-making.

2. **Understand your numbers:** Develop a comprehensive understanding of your business's financial landscape. Each and every financial metric—revenues, expenses, balance sheets, cash flows—holds significance. Hire the correct financial, tax, insurance, and legal advisors to help you understand the details.

3. **Revamp accounting and bookkeeping:** Overhaul your existing accounting and bookkeeping systems for improved accuracy and transparency. Solid and reliable financial records are the backbone of informed planning and decision-making.

4. **Evaluate your team:** Conduct a thorough assessment of your team's competence, commitment, and effectiveness. It's essential to maintain a team that resonates with the company's mission, driving it toward success.

5. **Restructure management:** If necessary, reconstruct your management team. Strong and effective leadership is key to fostering productivity and encouraging progress.

6. **Review and revamp SOPs:** Examine your current Standard Operating Procedures (SOPs) for their effectiveness and alignment with your business goals. Based on this evaluation, streamline and revamp the SOPs to ensure operational efficiency, reduce errors, and provide clear, actionable guidelines for your team.

7. **Monitor performance and ensure accountability:** Establish a system for regular monitoring of business performance and individual accountability. This helps track progress, identify areas for improvement, and ensure that everyone is contributing to the company's success.

By methodically following these steps, you are better equipped to proactively address and rectify issues, implement necessary changes, and steadily guide your business back onto the path of profitability. These steps operate in perfect harmony with the 7-28 Method.

My initial intuition had led me astray in my business, but the harsh lesson taught me to be more discerning and vigilant in my dealings. Now, I rely on my intuition to set off a siren as soon as something is wrong or if there's something I overlooked. It's vital to remember that intuition is not an infallible magic wand but a guide. It is a voice that we must respect and nurture, learning to distinguish its wisdom from the noise of our fears and insecurities. We must understand how to engage it and allow it to work alongside our logical minds to form an integral part of our decision-making arsenal. When we invite our intuition into the boardroom of our decisions, it will invariably help us navigate the dynamic and uncertain terrains we often encounter.

So, how do we tune into this frequency more effectively, especially when meeting new people in life or business? It begins with "qualifying" these individuals. As a professional, you should consider asking questions such as:

- What are their key goals?
- What does success look like for them?
- What are their challenges or pain points?
- How did they handle a past project's failure or success?

And on a more personal level, you may want to inquire:

- What are their values?
- What are their hobbies and interests?
- What experiences shaped who they are today?
- How do they handle conflict or adversity?

These questions are not meant to interrogate but to provide a clearer understanding of who they are. This will, in turn, help your intuition form a more accurate picture. According to Jack Welch, the well-known CEO of GE, a company is often comprised of 20 percent "A players," with 70 percent being "B players," and the remaining 10 percent being "C players." Welch had a practice of letting go of the lowest performing 10 percent of his workforce, which he deemed the "C players." His intuition told him that this approach would elevate overall performance by making space for more capable employees.[8]

Remember, intuition isn't about jumping to conclusions but about absorbing the subtle clues and nudges that enable us to make more informed decisions. It is our silent partner that helps us steer our ship in the right direction, especially when the waters are choppy. Through practice, we can all learn to listen better to this inner voice and leverage its power for personal and professional growth.

## DODGE THE PITFALLS: KNOW THE CHALLENGES IN YOUR PATH

Striking the right balance between risk tolerance and risk capacity is vital for anyone looking to steer clear of becoming another cautionary tale. You need to discern the level of risk you're comfortable with while also understanding the calculated risks you must take to succeed. In any endeavor, knowing your own metrics and understanding potential pitfalls are crucial for informed decision-making.

Consider this sobering statistic: according to data from the Bureau of Labor Statistics, as cited by Fundera, approximately 20 percent of small businesses don't make it past the first year. By the fifth year, that failure rate jumps to 45 percent, and by the 10th year, a staggering 65 percent of small businesses have closed their doors.[9] These numbers emphasize the need for acute awareness and proactive planning.

Let's discuss the five most common challenges that business owners face, based on my own observations:

1. They have a vision but not a process.

2. They hire people who are just like them (instead of finding people who fill their knowledge gaps).

3. They're too busy to train the people who come on board.

4. They hire people too quickly and take too long to fire the wrong ones.

5. They leverage themselves the wrong way, mentally, physically, and monetarily.

The riskiest type of business owner is one who has all motivation and zero consistency. Many goals, from a dream vacation to financial security, are achievable with a well-defined plan. The challenge lies in execution. By approaching life with a strategic framework, you improve your chances of achieving meaningful goals while also making room for happiness and fulfillment. Remember, no goal is insurmountable when you break it down into manageable pieces and commit to consistent progress. So, embrace the power of setting achievable targets and witness the transformation in your life.

## METRICS FOR MASTERY: BREAKING DOWN THE WORK

As we wrap up this chapter, let's not forget that even a boss has to monitor performance. Breaking down work into quantifiable goals is how you measure the progress you make in your life. Embracing the "work smarter, not harder" philosophy is a must for business owners with aspirations of substantial success. Assume you own a consulting firm that aims for $500,000 in annual revenue. With services priced at $5,000 per project, you'd need to complete 100 projects in a year. To scale, consider offering monthly retainers. With 20 clients at $2,500 per month, you'd generate $600,000 annually, exceeding your initial goal and creating residual income. If your services cost $25,000 per client, you'd only need three to four clients a month to reach the next potential goal of $1 million in gross annual revenue.

Setting goals requires balance. Aim too high and risk discouragement; aim too low and settle for mediocrity. It's common for business owners to build skyscrapers of goals. That's an intimidating climb. The hardest skill to learn is getting the goalpost to stop moving. Grant Cardone's 10X mindset is a popular approach, but let's face it—setting out-of-this-world goals doesn't always work for everyone. Here is my CliffsNotes version of his approach so you can see if it's a good fit for you: set targets that are 10 times greater than what you believe you can achieve, and take actions that are 10 times greater than what you think is necessary. And if you're into that strategy, check out *The 10X Rule* by Grant

Cardone, a motivational audiobook (also available as a paperback) that I've listened to dozens of times.[10] It's still about pushing yourself without risking burnout or bankruptcy!

There are many approaches out there—the 10X Rule, 7-28 Method, A.C.H.I.E.V.E—and while not all of these might work for everyone, there's definitely one out there that can take you to the top. Find that approach. Work on it daily. Integrate it into every single thing you do. And before you know it, you'll be shaking hands with your inner Boss.

"Who wants to be average?"

—Grant Cardone

# 06

# The Art of Effective Communication

Now that you've learned how to spot and dismantle invisible barriers in your way, how to set goals, and how to motivate yourself like you're Will Smith in *The Pursuit of Happyness*, it's time for us to dive into the world of echoes and effective communication. The universe has a funny way of testing us, doesn't it? Just when you start feeling like you've got your life, love, or finances in order—bam!—something comes out of nowhere, trying to throw a wrench in your plans. It's a classic case of "two steps forward, one step back." You're there, confidently strutting through life, thinking, "Hey, I've got this 7-28 Method thing down." But oh no, life says, "Hold my coffee." Suddenly, obstacles appear like surprise party crashers, determined to mess up your carefully crafted game plan.

In a world where the media seems bent on shouting, tweeting, and flashing news into your ears, eyes, and even dreams (I'm looking at you, pop-up ads), it can feel like you're swimming in a sea of ceaseless echoes. As much as you need to understand these echoes, you also need to know how to resist and respond to them. Fear not! This chapter is your trusty lifeboat, teaching you to distinguish your authentic voice from the media's surround sound system. I'll show you how to supercharge your voice, boosting its strength, volume, and resonance.

# RESISTING ECHOES: COUNTERING NEGATIVE MEDIA INFLUENCE

I have spent a good portion of my life listening to and following the echoes; I believed the narrative that the world was out to get me. I clung to every new echo that supported my victim mindset.

Take the media as an example. Tune into the news, and it's a 30-minute segment divided between three minutes of heartwarming stories and 27 minutes of horror stories. Fear, anger, uncertainty—these emotional buttons are pushed, pressed, and prodded. It's wave after wave of high-emotion echoes. For the average viewer, watching anything nowadays leaves you wildly confused, sad, or angry, depending on what and when you are watching. Just like reality shows bank on love and life woes, CNBC's expert panel is there to squabble over your financial forecast. Ever wonder why there's always a motley crew of contrasting opinions on these shows? Because disagreement keeps the viewer glued to the screen. The shows offer waves of negative vibrations from the echoes they project; many of us find comfort in this familiarity, regardless of the possibly depressing content. That noise consumes our minds, fertilizing the garden of our worst thoughts and watering our issues until they bloom into full-blown problems. And it's time for an intervention. I'm not saying ignore news updates entirely. Just be mindful of what you're consuming. If you struggle with a positive mindset, don't sandbag it with further negativity.

Dale Carnegie suggests the "zip it" approach, telling us to never criticize, complain, or judge (condemn) others.[11] It sounds easy, but when I started to follow these rules, I saw how often I was actually doing the opposite. Changing these habits became a tough challenge. Good communication starts with how you talk to yourself, and then you expand it out to others. You can't change how other people act, but you *can* change how you respond to them. Following the "zip it" idea helped me focus more on keeping a positive attitude. I started only worrying about what I could control in any situation. And this approach can do the same for you.

Once I started consciously changing my outlook, I began to recognize the negative messages that media spreads and the negativity others seem to carry. It was a wake-up call for changing my mindset, and one particular conversation revealed to me how talking negatively is often an unconscious reflex for some people.

One day, a family member called me, immediately launching into a barrage of complaints the moment I answered the phone. Spotting a rare break in the monologue, I chimed in, "Can you share three good things that happened to you today?"

Her shocked silence was followed by a struggle to answer and ended with a sarcastic, "Not everything is rainbows and unicorns, Amanda." That was telling enough. It wasn't surprising though, considering she was a devoted fan of daytime TV and news broadcasts. The drama and showmanship are a far cry from genuine emotion, and they can completely inhibit your ability to communicate effectively.

# IMPLEMENTING THE THREE Cs TO SPUR GROWTH

For someone to condemn or criticize my spirit, work ethic, drive, or purpose shows me that it's their issue, not mine. I used to take it personally and tell myself, "Maybe I *do* work too much. Maybe I *do* come on too strong." You can burn your energy focusing on what other people think of you or how they might perceive you, or you can channel your self-truth. For me, that means saying, "I am my own Boss. I'm being assertive. I'm in control, and I'm setting healthy boundaries for myself." If you're thinking of yourself as bossy, then you're listening to somebody else's view of you and repeating their perception as if it's the truth. Relying on others to validate you puts your self-esteem beyond your control and perpetuates feelings of insecurity. If this is an area you struggle with, seek out resources to help you.

I remember the first time I heard Gary Vee. I tuned into his podcast, and that one move was a total life-changer. Gary emphasizes self-awareness, hustle, empathy, and patience as keys to success, and his messages are tailored to motivate and inspire his audience to take action in their lives. Think of him like Tony Robbins, but he says the f-word a lot. He cuts right through the BS noise and says what he's thinking. He has the ideal story, having started a business from nothing. I have probably learned more eye-opening things from listening to Gary Vee than I have from any other person I've ever listened to. He's an incredible communicator, sharing what he thinks and discussing his experiences.

His podcast was like hearing all the tiny voices in my head out loud for the first time. He gave me a light so I could see, just like he has given to millions of others. I was letting people influence my mindset and rent space in my head, and *I* was paying for it! He helped me realize that self-doubt needs to go out the window to make space for self-evolution. You have to own who you are and practice being confident every day.

If there was a pill you could safely take to make everything perfect, then everyone would pop it. But a worthwhile life isn't so easy. It's the grind and daily conditioning that create sustainable changes. Just as going to the gym isn't a one-time effort, you can't give yourself one pep talk and expect real changes. It's a battle of you against you for your entire life, and you have to know how to win that battle. For me, replacing the three Cs—condemning, criticizing, and complaining—with three alternative tactics has made a significant difference:

1. **Shift from *criticizing* to constructive feedback:** Instead of pointing out flaws, offer positive suggestions.
   - *Example*: Instead of saying, "This report is full of errors," you could say, "Here are a couple of points that you might need to revisit for clarity."
   - *Example*: Replace your remark of "This design isn't good," with a suggestion: "How about we incorporate this color or element for better impact?"

2. **Replace *condemning* with curiosity:** Swap snap judgments with open-ended questions to gain understanding.

   - *Example*: Rather than declaring, "You're always late," ask, "Is there something that's making it hard for you to get here on time?"
   - *Example*: Substitute a statement of "This method is wrong," with an inquiry: "Can you walk me through your thought process on this?"

3. **Substitute *complaining* with your commitment to change:** Set personal goals to redirect focus from what's going wrong to what you can proactively change.

   - *Example*: Instead of lamenting, "I'm always so tired in the mornings," set a goal to go to sleep an hour earlier.
   - *Example*: Rather than griping, "I never have time for hobbies," commit to setting aside 30 minutes a week for a personal activity.

They sound simple and almost inconsequential, but I can guarantee that many of you, like me, tend to have knee-jerk reactions to situations. We instinctively open our mouths to condemn, criticize, or complain without our thoughts even catching up. This becomes such a big part of your routine that it's almost second nature. This is why some people stay in relationships, continue in unfulfilling jobs, or maintain poor eating habits—there's a sense of comfort they have adapted to. Remember, the *dis*comfort zone? Routine, even if it's negative, is everyone's default backslide. I've been there. There have been times when all I wanted to do was condemn or complain or criticize—these had become my solution, my own twisted form of therapy. I would often vent to my friends, followed by a glass of wine before bed, only to repeat the cycle the following day.

I've found out that breaking this cycle is a long, tiring process of setting goals and working hard to keep up with them while trying not to slip back into the toxic patterns you've gotten used to. You can start with a basic goal. Dedicate one day or even a few minutes to a simple exercise. Take a piece of paper, draw three columns, and in each, write the words "condemn," "criticize," and "complain." Under each word, note all of the different ways you do this and how often. You may start to see a pattern of what or who provokes you to instigate negativity, and this understanding could be your catalyst to make some serious lifestyle changes.

## TIMING IS EVERYTHING (ESPECIALLY WHEN COMMUNICATING)

You may have noticed that when your job or another part of your life hits the stress accelerator, you kind of become a carrier pigeon, delivering that energy back to your home. While it's easy to divide task lists, it's much harder for us to compartmentalize emotions. I've become hyper-aware of the emotional baggage I lug around from past experiences and how it's become an unwanted party crasher in my interactions. I swear Miranda Lambert's song "Baggage Claim" took on a whole new meaning after my deep dive into self-awareness. To communicate with finesse, you need to unpack and inventory your emotional suitcase before you can even think about sprucing up the conversation part. Think about the last handful of arguments you've been part of:

- Who played the other half of the duet?
- What were you arguing over?
- What was the cause?
- How did the dust settle?
- Could you have navigated these rapids differently?

People often find it tough to wade through these queries solo. I did the preliminary legwork myself and then brought in the big guns—my resources, spanning from my therapist to a business podcast. Scouting a resource that aligns with your self-evolution journey is vital, and it's doubly essential to let that resource nudge you to achieve a fresh perspective of yourself.

From my experiences in previous and current relationships, I've deduced that one of the key aspects of communication is understanding how to disagree with your partner effectively. This doesn't mean that conflict should be the dominant mode of interaction, but rather, it acknowledges that for many of us, anger is a manifestation of deeper issues, a symptom. The intensity of this symptom can make it very challenging when situations do not unfold as we desire them to. Sometimes, in our eagerness to have things play out exactly right, we force communication at an inopportune time. Choosing the right moment for a heart-to-heart is as equally important as knowing how to respectfully and effectively disagree.

It's as important as a comedian's punchline timing. Too early and the laughter is prematurely quelled. Too late and you'll lose your audience. You need to carefully select the perfect moment to raise a topic; nudge your partner, friend, family member, etc. to mull over something new; or kick-start a conversation that could be a stress bomb for both of you. If you bring up something at the wrong time, like when they're tired to the bone after a long day of work, one wrong comment could really set them off. So, when I have something I need to hash out with my hubby, I respect his emotional territory and state of mind. I specifically ask, "When do you think you'll be in the right headspace for this chat?"

Now, he playfully responds, "Check back in three months, dear," although he usually circles back within 15–30 minutes, and I reciprocate.

This approach is more productive than exploding emotions at each other. Be aware and respectful of how the person you're talking to is feeling, what their emotional levels are, and the time—this can help you gauge how productive or disruptive the conversation can be. Based on this assessment, you can adapt the conversation to work better for both of you. Read the room, and be sure to communicate effectively.

# BECOMING SELF-AWARE OF YOUR TALKING PATTERNS

So much of communication is recognizing our own baggage. Try as we might, the way we speak often acts as a projector, casting our internal feelings onto the external realm. In the past, I found myself perpetually defensive. Any time I established a boundary or encountered criticism, I felt the need to justify and explain. This reflex stemmed from an inner fear of inadequacy. I was communicating out of fear instead of truth. The reality is that we don't need to defend our worth, our truths, or our aspirations.

The truth is self-assured and holds firm even when questioned. Don't let your communication waver under scrutiny, or you'll end up distorting the truth. This used to be a familiar routine in my talking patterns. I was continuously people-pleasing, even if it meant I strayed away from the truth. And it was a disaster. It helped me realize that we only truly evolve spiritually when we master the art of honest communication, genuine apologies, and unblinking self-accountability.

As we heal and gain self-trust, the compulsion to over-explain or defend diminishes. Genuine confidence isn't boisterous; it resides in silence. As challenging as it is, don't let external perceptions sway the way you engage with the world. External challenges should not undermine you; they should ignite the fierce Boss within. Here are a few anchoring thoughts for moments when you're tempted to over-justify and fall into fruitless talking patterns:

- **Boundaries are your prerogative:** If someone tries to guilt or shame you for them, recognize it as their personal struggle and do not cave. You have every right to protect yourself and understand your limits.

- **Your truths are irrefutable:** Your experiences and feelings hold weight. Respect these truths.

- **Remember, it's human nature to project:** Often, when people project their insecurities or unresolved issues, it's more about them than you. Choose to create a space for healthy communication or take leave of the situation.

- **Give yourself the gift of self-compassion:** Sometimes, the wounds of our inner child can resurface, causing us to react based on past traumas. Recognize it, and treat yourself with grace.

Reminding yourself of these four thoughts can help you communicate more effectively and confidently. When you do get the opportunity to use that beautiful, strong voice you are growing, how does it sound? Have you ever found yourself tallying the number of filler words like "um," "uh," "like," "actually," and "you know" that someone uses in conversation? It's surprising how quickly these verbal hiccups can accumulate. Perhaps you're guilty of these same conversational patterns. My initiation into the world of radio broadcasting came with a stark realization of my rapid speech pace, something I was initially oblivious to. During my debut show, anxiety got the better of me. I had meticulously prepared ten pages of content, only to find myself scrambling for words just 15 minutes into a half-hour show. As confident as I was in the topic, I was totally thrown off my game.

In the grip of panic, my co-host, Marc Bernier, emerged as my saving grace. He expertly filled the ensuing silence and set me up with a few straightforward questions to navigate through the remaining airtime. This experience introduced me to the rhythm and tempo of my voice, a vital lesson taught to me by Marc and refined by one of my coaches. Marc was a giant in the radio industry, renowned for his skill and experience. He was more than a colleague, transforming into a cherished friend up until his unfortunate passing from COVID in August 2021. Marc's belief in my potential, his constant encouragement, and his genuine celebration of my successes pushed me to do and be better.

Mastering the cadence of your voice is about more than just modulating your pitch and pace; it's also about expressing your thoughts in a clear and self-assured way. Here are a few practical tips to help you achieve this:

- **Active listening:** Observe skilled speakers and dissect what makes their speeches so compelling. Using their rhythm and intentional pauses to emphasize keywords and tonal variation, attempt to adopt these traits into your speech.
- **Self-recording:** Recording yourself is another powerful tool for improvement. Listen or watch the playback of your voice and movements,

focusing not only on the physical presence of yourself but also the content of your speech, specifically on the filler words, pacing, and tone. You'll be surprised by how many filler words and unnecessary phrases you use or how often you might unconsciously shift your tone, pace, and movement. Note these moments and work on reducing them in your next practice sessions.

- **Visual cues:** Implement visual aids like a tally counter to monitor your usage of filler words. With deliberate practice, you'll gradually see a reduction in their frequency and a boost in the cadence of your speech.

- **Physical movements:** Pay attention to any physical cues you naturally resort to when speaking. Many people rock or bounce when speaking or use their hands like they are throwing confetti. Others rely on facial expressions to further convey their message. If you're hosting a podcast, remember those cues aren't effectively communicated over audio. Instead, try mirroring these cues in your vocal inflections instead. For example, if raising your eyebrows is your go-to sign of surprise, aim to express that surprise vocally instead. Now, for those who've discovered the fountain of youth through Botox, don't worry about the eyebrow trick; it's off the table anyway!

Regular practice incorporating these strategies, combined with ongoing self-assessment, can significantly improve the quality and rhythm of your speech. Remember, your voice is your instrument in radio or podcasts—learning to play it well will make all the difference in captivating your audience. If I had never met Marc, I would have gone through life speaking as if I was trying to win a speed race. He taught me to slow down, speak clearly and passionately, and communicate in a way that people will actually listen. That makes the difference between what is said versus what message is received.

## KEEP CALM AND COMMUNICATE

I don't expect you to turn around and become an expert speaker. But as a reader of this book, you're on the road to self-improvement, and communication is a vital part of that progress. Avoid the pitfalls of condemning, criticizing, and complaining. Instead, find ways to positively connect with your environment. In your role as leader, be clear in your expectations and support your team through praise. Gary Vaynerchuk once said, "Success is not just about making money. It's about making a difference."[12] With that in mind, go forth and effectively use that power.

# 07

# Visualizing and Manifesting Your Inner Dynamo

As a kid, I was convinced my superpower was speed. I was playing all sorts of sports, oftentimes with only boys on the field. My dad was always pushing me to run harder and faster and eat up the earth with my legs. I was just as strong emotionally, even then. People would call me "Demanda." I was bossy, stubborn, and as many would say, unyielding. Nowadays, qualities like kindness, empathy, intelligence, listening, and an unwavering focus on being interest**ed** instead of interest**ing** have provided a new path to achieving my goals. I work tirelessly, approaching tasks with the fierce determination of a lion—or rather, a lioness.

The qualities that have made me so successful often go unnoticed or unappreciated, especially in the intensely competitive world of finance, my chosen profession. The industry is notorious for its self-centered mindset—a discomforting thought that has always felt like a pebble in my shoe. Instead, I've spent my career making financial literacy accessible and building meaningful relationships through attentive listening. I prioritize my clients' needs and invest in them above all else, setting myself apart as an "exception" in this competitive—often self-serving—field.

In meetings, clients bring their fears and concerns, and I use my superpowers to dissect and understand their unique financial needs. Take one of my clients, Charly, for instance. She's been with me for 18 years, which is an eternity in the financial world. Although her account size may not be substantial, the trust and mutual growth she has offered are priceless. It was my distinct blend of compassion and empathy that appealed to Charly, and in turn, she helped shape me into the empathetic advisor I am today.

Your superpowers are not always traits that come naturally. One of my other superpowers was something I had to work hard on; forgiveness took me a while to cultivate. In moments of trauma, I clung to grudges and made selfish decisions. It was easy to blame my parents for every shortcoming I had. Over time, I've learned the transformative power of forgiveness. It hasn't been easy, but it's a necessary journey. By understanding my parents, their limitations, and their experiences, I began to understand them. We tend to put our parents on a pedestal and judge them harshly for any flaws or mistakes. Instead, I learned to humanize them, which allowed me to release anger and frustration. And forgiveness may follow further down the path.

Forgiveness (or your specific superpower) cannot be mastered overnight! I needed help to access mine. A lot of help. The first step was reaching out to others to find that support. Seek support, study gratitude, challenge negativity, and be the master of your transformation. Embrace your superpowers, knowing that personal growth is within your grasp. Alongside your arsenal of superpowers, you need to create a mindset of success. One that leads to prosperity in every sphere of your life.

## ASK, BELIEVE, RECEIVE

To make long-lasting, impactful changes to your mindset, you need to tap into your internal strengths and motivations. Developing superpowers or shifting your mindset is more than just being aware of the changes you need to make—you also need to practice them. Over time, I've developed a kind of mantra to help me deal with situations on the daily. It's not a direct means to your end but is a rallying cry of sorts to help you on your intensive journey toward growth.

The more positive mantras you take in, the more positivity you'll be bringing to your perspectives. It may not be a magic spell that will get you what you want, but it will prepare your mindset to *ask* for what you want and need and *believe* you deserve to *receive* it.

Recently, I applied the "Ask, Believe, Receive" strategy for it to not rain on my wedding day. I know it sounds like a fanciful gamble, but hear me out. I took this approach: "Sure, we'll take precautions and put down a deposit on tents, just to be on the safe side. But let's try this out. Let's 'Ask, Believe, and Receive' for clear skies." Remarkably, on October 22, 2022, the skies above Lisbon, Ohio, didn't have a single cloud! Call it luck or the power of this manifestation; either way, the tents were superfluous and my wedding day was gorgeous.

And when "Ask, Believe, Receive" doesn't come through, I no longer ask, "Why?" I ask, "What can I learn from this?" Sometimes, it means that there's something more I have to learn. I may have to go through an experience to get out on the other side of it. And that's okay. Progress takes time.

Not so long ago, I had a friend named Alex who was mulling over a significant career pivot. Encased in doubt, Alex nevertheless plucked up the courage to go on job interviews. One opportunity offered him an annual salary of $80,000. Seeing room for negotiation, I suggested, "Ask, Believe, Receive! The worst outcome is a no, but you'll never find out unless you make the ask." In spite of some initial apprehension, Alex requested a higher salary—a bold leap to $100,000 a year. The company came back with a counteroffer of $92,000 annually, a substantial raise from their initial offer. Alex was not only taken aback but also deeply motivated. This negotiation led to a yearly increase of $12,000, prompting Alex to think over the potential changes this could bring to his lifestyle. I urged him to consider the overall impact of this new position on his life rather than focusing solely on the financial uplift. By challenging his limits, Alex managed to secure what he truly deserved, leading to a significant boost in his self-confidence. This experience demonstrated the power of *asking* for what you're worth, *believing* in your value, and being open to *receiving* it.

Embracing the mantra "Ask, Believe, Receive" not only instills positivity in you amidst uncertain circumstances, but it also empowers you to envision multiple outcomes. Many people spend a portion of their day worrying about things that have very low probabilities of even happening. Rather than fretting about an unforeseen event or devoting energy to anxious thoughts, my approach lets you explore potential responses to different scenarios in advance. It's not about expecting the worst; it's about embracing adaptability and being ready for whatever life throws at you. Take for instance, my wedding; while I had applied the "Ask, Believe, Receive" strategy for it to not rain, I still had a contingency plan in mind. If a freak storm appeared out of the blue, I was ready to say, "Alright, let's set up the tents and adjust the layout, problem solved!"

Discussing alternatives doesn't mean they'll happen, but having considered them reduces their magnitude in your mind, allowing you to react with ease if they do occur. I see this as one of my newfound abilities: the knack to manifest what I desire from life. Harnessing the strength of our minds to shift our perspective and to seek positivity brings noticeable differences in our decision-making processes. Gone are the days where I stew in negativity—I played that tune in my 20s, and now it's time for a new beat. That leads me to another crucial pillar, that of having the self-awareness to unleash your inner dynamo.

## GAINING SELF-AWARENESS

You need to know *yourself*. To begin to tap into your superpowers and manifest your goals for yourself, first take stock of who you are and how you need to evolve. Start with your daily life outside of work. What energy are you putting out? How do you engage with others? Are you generally satisfied with your day? Why or why not? I can't offer a switch that will make every day perfect, but

I can help you find the awareness to make the necessary changes.

Then, let's shift to who you are in the professional world. How are you being perceived? How are you approaching your career tasks and goals?

During my extensive work with entrepreneurs, I've made keen observations, uncovering ways to unleash growth potential. It's not about doing it all yourself; it's about inspiring and attracting the right people and cultivating a positive energy that fosters personal growth and fulfillment. It's about practicing awareness in the moment, when barriers fall away and clarity emerges, transforming fear into a path of unlimited possibilities. Through my explorations of various training programs and devouring countless books, I've managed to uncover a categorization system to help you unleash your growth potential and channel your manifestation energy in the right direction.

One crucial element of gaining awareness is figuring out the type of person you are. For example, bosses often align themselves with Les McKeown's four leadership personality styles in his book, *Predictable Success*.[13] They are as follows: The Visionary, The Operator, The Processor, and The Synergist. Each personality carries unique strengths and challenges.

- **The Visionary:** Visionaries are big-picture thinkers, brimming with ideas and loaded with charisma. They are driven by possibilities and innovation, often becoming the catalysts for new projects and change in organizations.

- **The Operator:** Operators are action-oriented individuals who excel at getting things done. They are decisive and pragmatic and aren't afraid to roll up their sleeves to solve problems and achieve goals.

- **The Processor:** Processors are detail-oriented and thrive on structure, systems, and processes. They value consistency and predictability and are crucial for scaling and managing complexity within organizations.

- **The Synergist:** Synergists are the glue that holds the team together, and they excel in interpersonal relationships, understanding, and managing team dynamics. They are effective at promoting cooperation and harmony within the team.

Reflect on which style you align with the most. Does this leadership personality style complement your unique superpowers? Do you need to develop a superpower to become the type of leader you want to be? It's important to note that these personalities aren't rigid, and leaders often develop different traits from each of these styles. As you explore these styles in your life, be sure you don't let them overwhelm your personality. If you're not careful, you'll start to carry over an attitude or behavior traits that are better left behind in the workplace. These attitudes can be grouped into four categories:

1. **The Burn Out:** You become uncaring and complacent and are constantly searching for "new tricks."

2. **The Worker:** You take being a "hands-on boss" too seriously, becoming another employee, not the employer.

3. **The Imposter:** You hype up everyone and hope things will work out but have no clue what it actually takes to scale and optimize your team.

4. **The Fire Station:** You're preoccupied, busy putting out fires instead of creating systems. It becomes a tradeoff of health for wealth.

Now, if you find yourself resonating with one or more of these attitudes, professionally or even in your personal life, you'll likely catch yourself uttering some familiar phrases:

- "I don't have enough time."
- "I can't find the right people."
- "I can't afford staff."
- "It's easier to do it myself."

If any of these thoughts or emotions resonate with you, take comfort—you're not alone in this journey! Once we recognize and define the situations that occur in each sphere, it allows us to determine how to fix them and who can help us.

We're social beings, so it's natural to lean on others for support. At the same time, you have to be sure not to let other people's wants and preferences overpower your own. It's human nature to "run with the pack," and we're often persuaded to compromise and accept the status quo. Don't get swept away. I've been down that path—and trust me, it's fruitless. Instead, tap into your superpowers. You can use it to harness your fortitude to conquer any unsettling, daunting, or challenging situations. What differentiates me shouldn't be that I'm a particular demographic but that I apply my inherent superpowers: empathy, compassion, and listening. These traits have served me well in every successful personal and professional situation that comes to mind. When I'm faced with risks and opportunities, I utilize my "Ask, Believe, Receive" strategy to clarify my thoughts and manifest my desires. This isn't about creating false hope; it's about manifesting the right opportunities that evolve from practicing my superpowers.

## MANIFESTING DIVINE CONNECTIONS

My best example of manifestation is my journey toward motherhood. I have put in years and years of work to build my net worth and my self-worth in defiance of society's playbook for little girls. But trust me, blocking out societal noise is harder than turning off a fire alarm. I did find a sweet spot as "AuntDa," a super cool, supportive aunt to my three nephews, a niece, and a handful of amazing kids from my friends. I was all set to walk down the AuntDa lane and thought motherhood missed my address. At 40, I felt at ease with not wearing all the hats, but deep down, I knew something was off. I couldn't pinpoint the problem and didn't fully understand how to resolve this. And it was clear that this feeling—whatever it was— would inhibit my growth. I mean, how could I endorse positivity and manifestation if I wasn't ready to walk the talk? So, I decided to seek help. Or rather, help found me.

By a stroke of luck, or perhaps the universe's mysterious ways, I crossed paths with a fantastic woman named Melody, an energy coach and healer. Highly recommended by another Boss, I reached out to meet her.

My first meeting with Melody was nothing less than transcendental, unimaginable, and awakening. Yes, it was all those things, and I mean them with sincerity. Melody gave me hope of a higher level of power within me. I started practicing manifestations with her about things I never thought were possible for me, like being a mom. Melody assisted me in forging a deeper connection with my inner energy and spirituality. Melody unveiled concepts such as "idea allergies" and "trapped emotions"—notions I was previously oblivious to but suspected were prevalent in my life. She guided me to let go of thoughts I was clinging to and to mitigate my negative energetic vibrations. Of course, this required effort, but it was by no means an insurmountable task. It began by being open to experimentation and by approaching the process with curiosity rather than caution. I cannot overemphasize the significance of readiness, willingness, and capability to embrace change when embarking on this energy path.

Four months later, my husband and I discovered that I was carrying our first child. The timing was movie-like perfect; we found out just a week before Christmas and joyfully spilled the beans to our family on Christmas Eve and Day. It felt nothing short of a Christmas miracle. I know this sounds crazy, but she was able to tell me the gender of my baby boy before I even got the results. Despite the heartache of my miscarriage at 12 weeks, my faith in the power of manifestation and energy healing remains unshaken. After all, the process affirmed its magic when I discovered I was pregnant. However, manifestation, as I've come to understand it, isn't just about the destination; it's also about the journey. The path is as crucial as the goal, and sometimes, the twists and turns we encounter have their own wisdom to impart. This is a process that will unquestionably push many beyond their customary comfort zones.

Drawing on the profound wisdom of Rumi, who said, "The wound is the place where the Light enters," the "Ask, Believe, Receive" strategy and the process of manifesting is about revealing your vulnerabilities, taking chances, and allowing growth and learning to illuminate your path.[14]

"The wound is the place where the Light enters."

—Rumi

# 08

# Sympathy vs. Empathy: Understanding Needs, Wants, and Pains

I had a coach say to me once, "The worst salespeople are the ones who only have a hammer, so they think that everything's a nail." I heard that years ago, and I still keep it in mind when I'm talking to others. Sure, you may have something important to say, but you can't just keep pushing it onto others. That mindset is what gives salespeople a bad name. You have to know when it's the right time to speak up and when it's best to stay quiet.

## CONNECTING THROUGH EMPATHY AND UNDERSTANDING

I've always loved talking to people, connecting, and making their dreams work. Even so, there have been instances when a dialogue quickly escalated into a dispute, leaving both parties frustrated. I finally had to admit the recurring issue was my manner of communication. No message, no matter how great, will get across if your delivery sucks. It was clear that I needed to change; I was determined to get better at communicating, in the professional world and personal settings.

Business success requires a two-way conversation, an exchange that goes beyond surface-level interactions to genuine understanding and assistance. It wasn't long before I saw that this principle held true not just in business but also in personal relationships. I observed that many people are hesitant to discuss their needs until they feel their underlying fears and pain points have been acknowledged. This realization led me to adopt a new method, the "pain pathway." Instead of merely sympathizing with the problems people faced, I worked on *empathizing* with them—putting myself in their shoes to better comprehend their concerns. After all, I knew we couldn't progress unless I removed the obstacles of pain blocking the path.

By adopting an empathetic approach, I could dig deeper into people's thoughts and emotions. This helped me identify their unique challenges and fears, enabling more productive conversations aimed at problem-solving. As we'll discuss later, advice on finances isn't all that different from guidance on relationships.

At times, communication with our partners is lacking no matter how sweet your relationship is. We tend to say little but expect a lot. It's part of human nature, but sometimes, we confuse what's being said versus what's being received. Whenever I start to react negatively to something someone has said, I ask myself, "Am I over-personalizing this?" And often, the answer is a yes.

If my partner or my client starts taking things a little too personally, or they begin to retreat into their shell instead of communicating, I dig deeper into their pain pathway by asking a series of probing questions using a "push-pull" approach; I push a client away so we can establish what the pain is. Essentially, I give them the space needed so we can have an open, straightforward, and productive discussion. Most salespeople are "pull" personalities, demanding answers and commitment from their clients. Knowing this, I walk through a mental script of questions to help me unravel my client's pain:

- What is their pain/fear?

- Where does it derive from?
- What would address it?

- What would reassure the client at that moment?
- What would make the pain feel lighter?

By taking the time to review these questions and connect with my clients, I can cater to more than just their financial concerns. Occasionally, I get stuck in an uncomfortable situation because I'm not telling people what they *want* to hear but rather what they *need* to hear. At times, when the dialogue begins to go downhill, I take a moment to recall a widely accepted truth in these situations: people often project their emotions (pains) and past experiences (more pain) onto present situations. They may retreat, but that's okay; I give them the space they need to confront reality and acknowledge and accept that there's value in what I'm telling them. For people who are resistant to the conversation, I look beyond their words to the source of their behavior (their pain point). It can often be attributed to:

- Their capability to manage their emotions;
- The communication methods instilled in them;
- The foundational beliefs they hold about themselves;
- Their self-view; or
- How they interpret the world, which is influenced by their past experiences.

In some instances, clients start to overlay their past negative encounters with other advisors onto *me*. They begin to interpret a simple piece of advice or question as a personal attack, thinking I'm pointing out their flaws when, in reality, I'm merely trying to assist them. It's in situations like these when it's most important to declutter the miscommunication and be direct. If something is misunderstood, it's instinctual to attack.

Culturally, we have a propensity to interpret other people's actions as direct reflections on us. This is misguided and shows how our ego is manifesting. Instead, this negative behavior often mirrors how they've been conditioned to be, working just like a projector. I look past this display to get to what my clients really need rather than what they're saying.

Sometimes, it takes everything in my power to breathe and not react. One prospective client came in and was immediately put off despite my warm demeanor. He said almost immediately that he didn't trust financial advisors (but still needed one). Many advisors would have shut down and given up on the whole meeting, but I knew there had to be a reason behind his statement. I couldn't help it; the quest was so intriguing to me.

"Okay, well, did something happen to you that caused you to develop this attitude? Tell me more," I asked him, trying to understand where he was coming from.

"My previous advisor lied to me," he said.

That wasn't entirely true: more of a miscommunication and lack of transparency on the advisor's part. This often happens in my field since financial products can be extremely detailed. There's a 50–500-page document that accompanies most products. Advisors like to give the CliffsNotes version, but I find most people don't even understand what they are buying. This confusion creates intense suspicion in the field, and that's why it's so important to pick a reputable advisor with lots of experience. I operate as a consultant, not a salesperson. You should feel very comfortable when working with a financial advisor and never feel put off or scared to ask questions. The relationship requires trust on both sides.

When a client expresses feeling betrayed by their previous advisor, it means I need to probe a little more to understand what really happened. So, I asked, "How could that situation have been handled differently for you not to have felt lied to?" It turns out that all he needed was to be walked through the paperwork and feel welcome to visit our office if he needed to ask a question. If I had reacted to his tone with judgment or if I launched criticism against the other advisor (which is what 95 percent of advisors do, leading to even more distrust with advisors), I wouldn't have seen the reason behind the fear. Instead, I led with empathy and was better for it. When you communicate clearly and calmly, it's human nature to reciprocate that behavior. I brought good energy into that meeting, and after addressing his concerns, he mirrored the same energy.

## USING YOUR VOICE WISELY

As I've grown to become more cognizant of people's feelings and their reactions to situations, one thing has always helped me get through to people: listening. When someone is vulnerable about their pains, they just want you to hear them out without judgment. They're searching for validation. Actively listen. Even when I'm not sure where a person is coming from, I simply ask questions and listen instead of assuming their intent. As Mark Twain famously said, "It is better to keep your mouth closed and let people think you are a fool than to open it and remove all doubt."[15]

By incorporating active listening and effective communication tools, I've noticed that my relationships are smoother. If my husband (or anyone) does or says something negative and my reflexive reaction is a resentful, "Get lost," I pause, count to five, and recite a calming mantra. With my husband, I think, *This person loves me. He doesn't want to hurt me. He's not trying to hurt me.* The sentiment can be modified for anyone, such as an employee: *This person depends on me. Are they trying to be mean to me, or do they just need direction, validation, or reassurance?*

Generally, the "formula" of the mantra can be thought of as answers to these questions:

- Is this directed toward me?
- Am I safe?
- What is this person hoping to achieve from what they're saying to me?

I reflect on where the other person is coming from and why my reaction is so visceral. Usually, I can identify the unspoken factors at play, but sometimes, I'm not so sure. I try to return with, "I'm a little confused," instead of ambushing with, "Why did you say that?" Speaking in a "you" language can feel like an attack, especially for those overwhelmed by their traumas, so I lean toward "I" statements instead. Or even better, focus on the team: "What can we do together to work on this?" I also like to offer a "menu" if they are at a loss for words. For example, "Usually when someone says this to me, it's because of A, B, or C. Do any of those resonate with you?"

The next step in successful communication is to apply this inner wisdom to the world around me. The lessons in this book are meant to teach you how to understand and heal yourself as well as guide you to connect with others in a meaningful way. It's not just about the messages we carry within but also the messages we send out— our timing, our voice. We often encounter moments when someone we care for is in a vulnerable state, expressing their pain or joy through tears, arguments, or celebrations. By distinguishing between sympathy and empathy, we can navigate these situations more skillfully. Sympathy might offer compassion, but empathy goes further, understanding the other person's pains, wants, and needs. How we respond can be a defining moment for that relationship.

"It is better to keep your mouth closed and let people think you are a fool than to open it and remove all doubt."

—Mark Twain

# FROM TEARS TO TRIUMPH

Throughout the stages of my life, my communication abilities varied immensely. Those skills grew as I grew *up*. My tears evolved, serving as barometers of my innermost feelings. In my early 20s, I found myself crying over seemingly trivial matters like my bank account balance or the inability to match a top to a pair of jeans. These tears were innocent, a direct response to immediate stressors. But as I matured into my 30s, my tears began to carry a deeper weight, revealing an inner complexity that I had not previously recognized. They were no longer merely reactions to external circumstances but resonating echoes of unresolved emotions and negative energy I had unwittingly harbored.

While relationships can be defined in moments of vulnerability and expression with each other, what happens when it's within yourself? How do you find a deeper way to address the issues inside you? I was still feeling the pains and pulls from my early traumas no matter how much positivity I consumed. Right after that second stern call from Ramey, I knew I could no longer handle this healing task all by myself. I had not yet crossed paths with Melody, so I began seeking guidance deeper than a traditional therapist. I wanted to consult someone who specialized in trauma. I needed more answers.

One of the most transformative therapies I engaged in was with Ed King, a trauma therapist who specializes in an exposure therapy called Traumatic Incident Reduction (TIR). This technique, which is intense but very effective, involved me confronting the traumatic incidents of my life by "viewing" them repeatedly in the safety of his office. Thus, eliminating their emotional hold on me. It's essential to understand that anxiety is a universal human emotion—feeling worry, fear, or apprehension about future events is completely normal. However, when this anxiety becomes excessive and persists, it evolves into an anxiety disorder, which can be crippling. These disorders, including generalized anxiety disorder, panic disorder, phobias, and social anxiety, are not uncommon as 4.7 percent of U.S. adults experience a panic disorder at some point in their lives. Symptoms can range from panic and fear to increased heart rate, rapid breathing, difficulty sleeping, nausea, and dizziness.[16] And if you or anyone you know has experienced these symptoms, you know firsthand how debilitating and limiting they can be. It was time for me to take charge of my trauma and improve my communication.

Besides TIR with Ed, I also utilized Eye Movement Desensitization and Reprocessing (EMDR), another potent form of psychotherapy.[17] During EMDR sessions, I was encouraged to recall past traumatic events while following specific eye movements, designed to stimulate the brain's natural healing process. Both TIR and EMDR are evidence-based treatments for conditions like anxiety disorders, proven to reduce symptoms and improve mental well-being. Had I not embarked on this transformative journey of self-discovery with my therapists—followed by the work I did with Ed—I doubt I would have been spiritually or emotionally prepared to absorb Melody's teachings just one year later. Maybe the universe itself wouldn't have aligned to place these healing opportunities in my path. I would encourage everyone suffering from psychological or emotional issues to contact a licensed therapist and see if either of these treatments would be appropriate for them. These treatments, among others, can be very powerful at releasing people from their past to attain their best future.

By consciously engaging with this inner landscape—the mountainous roads of my trauma—I laid the emotional groundwork that could sustain me in the future. When I faced my miscarriage, the support from Ed and Melody had already equipped me with resilience and deeper understanding. Though the pain was raw and devastating, the work I did in my late 30s allowed me to traverse this grief without succumbing to an overwhelming burden. My tears, once merely a response, had become a manifestation of my entire emotional journey.

Crying is nature's way of maintaining our emotional well-being. Laden with oxytocin and endorphins, tears activate our body's healing mechanism, steering us toward calmness and away from stress.[18] To suppress them is to deny ourselves the opportunity to heal. There is a time to grieve, to cleanse the soul of emotional toxins, but there is also a time to rise, to straighten your back, and to stride confidently into a future where personal well-being is paramount. As the Boss of my life, I choose to take charge and foster deep self-development.

Years ago, I could not have imagined possessing this progressive mindset and this level of emotional control. Just as I've advanced in my professional life—making modifications and becoming a better leader, manager, and teammate—I've learned to do the same in my relationships. My husband and I have been together for nearly a decade now, but we are vastly different from the people we were during the initial phase of our relationship. Had we remained unchanged, our relationship wouldn't have survived to the present day. Instead, we've developed and invested time and effort into ourselves and our relationship. We collaborate to enhance things. We've improved our communication, understanding, intimacy, finances, and even our professional endeavors. We genuinely acknowledge that while we are independent entities, we are more formidable as a unit. A Clydesdale can pull one-tenth its body weight on its own, but when you pair it with another Clydesdale, it can pull more than double the weight.

# 09

# Finances

Okay, Bosses! You're almost through this book. Great job! It's time to discuss the topic that has been the elephant in the room for centuries. Finances. For many, just the mention of this word is enough to send shivers down the spine. It's no wonder that the statistics related to it are staggeringly grim. Even our own nation seems to be wobbling under the weight of this overwhelming topic. Consider this: the gross national debt of America surpassed the unfathomable sum of $31 trillion in the third quarter of 2023, a first in U.S. history.[19] Let's pause. I need you to visualize this amount. Let's say I borrow $1 trillion that I have to pay back. How long would it take if I paid it back one dollar every second? Well, it would take 31,688 years to pay it back (and that's without interest)! Even in the face of our national debt, you're still expected to manage your money responsibly. And that's where we financial advisors come in.

Our fascination with money is so intense that since 1989, a clock has been ticking in Times Square, diligently tracking the U.S. national debt. Imagine if there was a clock of doom assigned to your finances or to your love life—how would you fare?

Every news item, no matter how seemingly unrelated, carries an undercurrent of financial implications. In fact, money is intricately woven into the fabric of our lives, touching every aspect we participate in. Yet, the widespread inclination is to avoid the subject as though it's a contagion. In the past, it was a commonplace notion to work until you died. This lingered until the late 70s. Roth IRAs did not even exist until 1998! In many ways, it's still a "new idea" to create a financial plan or have financial literacy. So, it's high time we shift our mindset. Understanding finances is not a burdensome chore; it's an empowering tool that can set us on a path to flourish. Money is not bad or good; it's just paper or numbers on a screen.

This subject is tackled toward the end of the book, not because it's less crucial but because it's essential to align your thinking patterns first. The idea is to ensure you are in the Boss mindset before setting out on your financial journey. Otherwise, you risk getting caught in the same cycle, repeating patterns in your life and relationships, and now in your finances. This is because not all financial fears are rational, and some fears are not even connected to the problem. Being a Boss of your finances requires getting a grip on the basics first, then building a strong understanding of financial principles, data analysis, strategic decision-making, communication, and collaboration. Developing these skills can take years of practice and requires a continuous effort to learn and improve. Getting good at this doesn't happen overnight. The financial world is constantly evolving, and it is essential to stay informed about the latest trends and best practices.

It's natural to feel overwhelmed by this topic. Maybe that's why you're here. Don't worry, one of my greatest passions is spreading financial literacy. I like to think of it as making finance fun, so keep reading! I remember feeling terrified when I entered the finance field at 23. However, I've learned over the years that effectively managing your finances is not just about having knowledge but also about developing a strong mindset and an impeccable team. It's essential to have confidence in your abilities and believe in your capacity to achieve goals. Embrace challenges as opportunities for growth, and don't be afraid to make mistakes—they are a requisite for learning and improving.

Whether your aspiration is to become a CERTIFIED FINANCIAL PLANNER™ (CFP®) like me, take charge of your personal finances, or interview advisors for help with your own planning and investments, having a fundamental understanding of money and the accompanying behaviors is crucial. First, we will explore the concept of money scripts and how they shape our beliefs and behaviors around money. Few people make financial decisions based on numbers or a spreadsheet. They are influenced by their friends, family, personal history, ego, pride, marketing, incentives, you name it—all of that is jumbled together into whatever script "works" for them. By gaining a baseline understanding of these scripts, we become empowered to understand what's driving us so we can make better financial decisions and create a healthier relationship with money.

## UNDERSTANDING YOUR MONEY SCRIPT

Understanding and working on your attitude toward building (or rebuilding) wealth is just as necessary as rejuvenating your body through adequate sleep, healthy eating, hydration, or cutting ties with toxic individuals. What good is wealth without health? Money scripts

 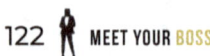

are deep-rooted beliefs about money that individuals develop, often originating from childhood experiences and influenced by family values. There is neuroscience on how we think, separated into our conscious and subconscious minds. The subconscious is a bit lazy though and designed not to work, however, that's where the bulk of our true beliefs lie. These subconscious ideas play a significant role in shaping a person's relationship with money throughout life.

Here are seven money scripts to consider:

1. **Money Avoidance:** Money Avoidance is a mindset where an individual equates money with discomfort or fear, often leading to neglect of their finances. For example, someone may avoid investing or doing financial planning because they feel overwhelmed by the financial decisions involved.

   *Tips to overcome Money Avoidance:*
   - **Break the tasks down:** Start with smaller, manageable financial tasks, and gradually take on more complex ones.
   - **Seek knowledge:** Regularly educate yourself about financial management, investments, and insurance to demystify the topics.
   - **Address the anxiety:** Identify and address the underlying fears or negative experiences related to money.

2. **Money Worship:** Money Worship implies a belief that accumulating wealth will solve all problems and bring happiness. An individual with this

script might overemphasize investing or buying expensive insurance policies, thinking more money equates to fewer problems.

*Tips to reduce Money Worship:*

- **Set balanced goals:** Cultivate financial goals that consider your happiness and well-being, not just your wealth accumulation.

- **Find joy in non-material things:** Explore happiness in relationships, hobbies, and personal development.

- **Reflect on financial decisions**: Regularly assess whether your financial choices align with your overall life values and goals.

3. **Money Vigilance:** Money Vigilance involves being extremely cautious and attentive with your money, perhaps avoiding risks associated with investments or always opting for the safest insurance policies. This might be due to fear of losing money or having financial instability.

*Tips to manage your Money Vigilance:*

- **Allow for enjoyable spending:** Dedicate a portion of your budget to personal enjoyment and fulfillment.

- **Assess risk tolerance:** Regularly review and understand your willingness to take financial risks.

- **Maintain an emergency fund:** Establish and maintain a fund for unexpected expenses to enhance financial security.

4. **Money Status:** Money Status is equating your worth with your financial status, possibly leading to overemphasis on wealth projection through investment portfolios or luxurious possessions. This can be driven by societal expectations or a desire for external validation.

*Tips to reduce your Money Status fixation*:

- **Cultivate internal worth:** Develop a sense of self-worth that is not reliant on financial status.
- **Live authentically:** Make financial decisions that are true to your values and needs, not to project an image.
- **Build real connections:** Develop relationships based on mutual respect and shared values rather than wealth.

5. **Money Dependency:** Money Dependency revolves around the belief in consistent financial rescue from others, leading to a potential reluctance to make independent investment or insurance decisions. This can stem from a lack of financial confidence or knowledge.

*Tips to mitigate your Money Dependency:*

- **Empower through education:** Learn about financial planning, investments, and insurance to make informed decisions.
- **Foster financial independence:** Work toward self-reliance through consistent income and responsible spending.

- **Set healthy boundaries:** Establish clear financial boundaries and expectations with others.

6. **Money Empowerment:** Money Empowerment is viewing money as a tool for personal growth and positive impact, influencing thoughtful investing and responsible insurance choices. This mindset often arises from an understanding of the potential benefits of responsible financial management.

*Tips to enhance your Money Empowerment:*

- **Align decisions with values:** Ensure that all financial choices reflect your core beliefs and goals.
- **Invest in personal growth:** Allocate financial resources to learning and self-improvement.
- **Create positive impact:** Utilize your finances to contribute to societal and environmental well-being.

7. **Money Balance:** Money Balance means valuing financial stability without letting it overshadow other life aspects. For instance, you might choose balanced investments and insurance that align with a holistic life approach, focusing on overall well-being.

*Tips to support Money Balance:*

- **Maintain life equilibrium:** Continually realign financial goals with broader life aspirations.

- **Practice intentional spending:** Make financial decisions thoughtfully, balancing various life priorities.

- **Develop adaptive strategies:** Learn to adapt your financial strategies to life's evolving circumstances.

Gaining insight into your money script is essential for evaluating your financial behavior and making informed decisions that will benefit your long-term financial well-being. If you recognize one of these money scripts, or perhaps several, as your go-to reaction when finances are brought up, be sure to unpack *why* you have such a strong response. How can you approach a financial advisor in such a way that your money script is addressed? If you find that there's so much built-up trauma that a trip to a financial advisor is petrifying, your first stop may need to be at a therapist or counselor's office. If you don't address your past, you can't plan for the future.

## Mindset Is Everything

Understanding and mastering your finances isn't merely a matter of calculations or budgeting; it's an introspective journey into your personal history, upbringing, beliefs, and emotions. To embark on this journey, start by visiting my site, www.aurionwealthadvisors.com, where you can take a quiz to identify the money script that resonates with you. This self-assessment tool helps shed light on the underlying beliefs and patterns that drive your financial behavior. Don't forget the workbook that accompanies this book, which is available at www.728method.com.

After you take the assessment, reflect on your childhood experiences with money. What were your parents' attitudes toward spending or saving? Was money a taboo subject, or were you encouraged to ask questions and understand it? Recall the details, such as the first toy or major purchase you desired and how you went about obtaining it; this journey through your memories can reveal valuable insights into your early formation of money-related values and habits.

Your financial mindset mirrors many aspects of your life and can be broadly categorized into two paradigms: scarcity or abundance. If you're dominated by anxiety, for example, you might have an underlying fear of losing control over your finances. Exposure to extravagant spending or secretive money habits during your childhood could create a pattern where you make financial decisions without fully weighing potential risks.

Working with clients, I've seen firsthand how these deep-seated beliefs influence financial behavior. Whether it's a substantial loss in the stock market or a previous negative financial advisory experience, understanding a client's unique mindset and history enables me to tailor solutions that address their specific concerns. By delving into their perceptions and asking for clarification on ambiguous terms, such as "a lot of money" or "a huge loss," I can align my assistance to fit their personal needs and beliefs. A surprising number of individuals wrestle with feelings of unworthiness regarding money. This internal strife can result in reckless spending or monetary hoarding behavior. Consider the fact that 70 percent of lottery winners lose their fortunes, according to the National Endowment for Financial Education.[20] Now contrast this with the self-made millionaires who demonstrate a cultivated ability to manage or delegate their wealth effectively. They appreciate the nuances of financial planning, allowing them to save and invest consistently, even after making a mistake and losing money.

Some people are self-starters and want to handle their finances all on their own. Others prefer to have an advisor help them manage both expected and unexpected life events. Regardless of preference, no one receives an expiration date on their birth certificate. Crafting a financial plan, either independently or with a professional, allows you to achieve peace of mind where you can be present for the people and moments that matter most in your life.

Your relationship with money is a complex, multifaceted reality of life. More than a matter of numbers, it's a reflection of who you are and how you were raised. By identifying your money script, reflecting on your history, and recognizing the psychological underpinnings, you can transform your relationship with money. This shift enables a more controlled, appreciative, and effective approach to your finances, leading to your long-term well-being and success.

## THE MAGIC OF COMPOUND INTEREST

Financial planning isn't just for the wealthy; you don't need millions to benefit from the guidance of experts in the field. In fact, the earlier you start planning and investing, the easier it is to achieve your financial goals. The longer you wait to start, the more difficult it becomes, and the larger the required amount is to reach your goals. That's why it's important to take advantage of the power of compound interest as early as possible. Every dollar you save and invest today has tremendous earning potential at a later date, and that potential can compound over time. But to benefit from this power, you need to be able to save up and invest consistently.

The Rule of 72 is a financial tool that can shed light on the transformative power of compound interest, especially for those who are in a position to invest beyond just saving for emergencies. If you're fortunate to have a job or run a business where you're earning more than just covering your basic needs and emergencies, understanding this principle can help you make informed decisions about your financial future.

Here's a simple breakdown.

The Rule of 72 calculates how long it'll take for your investment to double based on a given annual rate of return. You can divide 72 by your expected rate of return, and the result is approximately the number of years it'll take for your investment to double.

Let's say you're doing well in your career or business and decide to invest some of your earnings. If you expect a 10-percent annual return on your investment, using the Rule of 72, you'd compute:

$$72 \div 10 = 7.2$$

This means that with a 10-percent annual return, your investment would double in about 7.2 years.

To contextualize this with a real-world example, imagine you've done well in your job or business and can comfortably invest $50,000, expecting that 10-percent return. In just over seven years, that $50,000 would grow to $100,000. Thanks to compound interest, not only does your original amount earn interest, but the interest earns its own interest too!

Many of the clients I collaborate with on a one-on-one basis are positioned to make sizable annual investments. Consider Taylor, for instance. She's a business owner who just turned 48 and has a team exclusively made up of non-W-2 employees. (This distinction in employee classification is crucial for optimizing tax strategies.) Given the consistent profitability of her business, she's able to leverage a strategy I refer to as the "Pension Max Plan." Depending on the prevailing tax codes, she can invest up to $200,000 annually into this plan and simultaneously deduct this contribution from her adjusted gross income. This move yields her tax savings in excess of $75,000 each year. (Keep in mind, that's just one strategy a profitable business owner can use; we have several big-ticket savings strategies and vehicles for our clients. Chapter 10 discusses this some more).

Let's take a closer look at the numbers. If Taylor were to invest $200,000 annually for 16 consecutive years and earn an average return rate of nine percent, the Rule of 72 can give us some insights into her potential returns. By dividing 72 by 9, we get: 72 ÷ 9 = 8. This means her investments would approximately double in eight years.

To clarify, in the first eight years, Taylor's cumulative contribution of $1.6 million (eight years multiplied by $200,000) would be worth considerably more than just double due to the yearly additions and compound interest. However, for simplification: if she invests $200,000 in the first year, that specific amount might grow to around $400,000 by the eighth year. Then, by the 16th year, that initial $200,000 could potentially become $800,000 thanks to the compounding effect.

In reality, Taylor's overall portfolio value could be much higher due to her yearly contributions and the magic of compounding on the entire balance. In fact, over a 16-year period, Taylor's strategic investments using the Pension Max Plan would not only yield her a substantial sum of approximately $4,739,591.64, but she would also enjoy cumulative tax savings of $1,200,000. This showcases the dual benefits of her approach: significant growth in assets and substantial tax advantages, both accentuating the power of informed financial planning.

Let's move on to the next concept of investing. As I mentioned, it's never too late to start, but when you start will impact the math. Let's consider two investors: one is 25 and the other is 40. Say both individuals start with an initial investment of $5,000; the 25-year-old contributes $800 monthly, and the 40-year-old contributes $2,400 monthly. They both secure an eight percent annual return, compounded monthly.

# EXAMPLE 1

## INVESTING STARTING AT AGE 40

| Years of Investment | Age | Total Investment Value |
|---|---|---|
| 5 | 45 | $189,710 |
| 10 | 50 | $458,031 |
| 15 | 55 | $858,748 |
| 20 | 60 | $1,508,279 |

The first scenario is for a 40-year-old individual who earns $250,000 annually and aims to accumulate wealth until they turn 60. This person begins with an initial investment of $5,000 and commits to a monthly contribution of $2,400. They anticipate an 8% annual return, compounded monthly.

• Assumes a consistent 8% annual return, compounded monthly.
• Monthly contributions are made consistently at the beginning of each month.
• The final value is the total value of the investment at the end of the investment period, not adjusted for inflation.
• These examples are for illustrative purposes only and do not guarantee actual investment returns.

# EXAMPLE 2

## INVESTING STARTING AT AGE 25

| Years of Investment | Age | Total Investment Value |
|---|---|---|
| 10 | 35 | $144,731 |
| 20 | 45 | $460,905 |
| 30 | 55 | $1,166,783 |
| 35 | 60 | $1,830,238 |

The second scenario is for a 25-year-old individual who earns $75,000 annually and also aims to accumulate wealth until they turn 60. This person begins with the same initial investment of $5,000 and commits to a smaller monthly contribution of $800, while also expecting an 8% annual return, compounded monthly.

• Assumes a consistent 8% annual return, compounded monthly.
• Monthly contributions are made consistently at the beginning of each month.
• The final value is the total value of the investment at the end of the investment period, not adjusted for inflation.
• These examples are for illustrative purposes only and do not guarantee actual investment returns.

As evident from these tables, even though the 25-year-old is investing three times less per month than the 40-year-old, they end up with a larger total due to the power of compound interest over a longer period. This is a striking illustration of why starting early is a key strategy in wealth accumulation. If the 25-year-old in the example were to invest the same amount as the 40-year-old, using the same assumptions we started with, the 25-year-old would have accumulated $6,388,708.79 by 60. As you can see, with consistent monthly contributions and a long-term investment strategy, the individual would be well on their way to achieving their financial goals thanks to the power of compound interest stretched over a longer period of time. This example demonstrates the importance of starting early and sticking to a long-term investment strategy even if it means starting with smaller contributions.

Of course, it's important to keep in mind that investment returns are never guaranteed, and market fluctuations can impact the growth of your portfolio. These charts represent returns that are gross of fees. If you choose to work with an advisor or a CERTIFIED FINANCIAL PLANNER™, that could come with a cost, and that cost needs to be factored in when discussing overall returns. Be sure that whatever strategy you decide to go with you understand all costs involved.

## CONTROL YOUR NARRATIVE! BE YOUR OWN PERSONAL CHEERLEADER!

Our thoughts and beliefs about money can have a powerful impact on our financial success. In this section, we'll discuss seven simple money declarations that you can use to take charge of your finances. By making simple money declarations and regularly repeating them to ourselves, we can shift our mindset toward abundance and success.

The last time I was truly scared about my finances was when I opened my firm. My fear wasn't even rational at the time. I was ready to do it and had plenty of savings and financial stability, but I still felt a little like that terrified young lady who was told I wouldn't make it in finance, in "the boys' club." My firm became a reality, and during the pandemic, my business quadrupled in size. Yes, you read that right, an increase of *four times* my business and my earnings. It was incredible, and I attribute it to finally being my own Boss. I had the chance to finally tell that young lady, "You got this. You are the Boss of yourself, and everything you need to be successful is already inside of you. Just believe it!" I had jumped—no, leaped—and it was worth it.

Here are seven simple money declarations to help you take charge of your financial future:

- **"I am capable of managing my finances and achieving my financial goals."**
  - Believing in your ability to manage your finances is key to taking charge of your financial future. By regularly repeating this declaration to yourself, you can build confidence and trust in your abilities.
- **"I am worthy of financial abundance and success."**
  - Many of us have limiting beliefs about money and our worthiness. By affirming that you are worthy of financial abundance and success,

you can shift your mindset toward a more positive and abundant outlook.

- **"I am grateful for the money I have and for the opportunities to earn more."**
  - Practicing gratitude for the money you have, no matter how much or how little, can help you cultivate a positive mindset toward your finances. By focusing on abundance rather than scarcity, you can attract more opportunities for financial growth and success.

- **"I am in control of my spending and make wise financial decisions."**
  - Taking control of your spending and making wise financial decisions is key to achieving your financial goals. By affirming that you are in control of your spending habits, you can avoid impulse purchases and make intentional choices that align with your financial goals.

- **"I invest wisely and build wealth for my future."**
  - Investing wisely is an important part of building long-term wealth and achieving financial freedom. By affirming that you are a wise investor and are building wealth for your future, you can stay focused on your long-term financial goals.

- **"I am always learning and growing in my financial knowledge."**
  - Financial literacy is an ongoing process, and there is always more to learn. By affirming that

you are always learning and growing in your financial knowledge, you can stay engaged and informed about the latest trends and strategies for building wealth.

- **"I am open to opportunities for financial growth and success."**
  - Staying open to opportunities for financial growth and success can help you attract new possibilities and avenues for building wealth. By affirming that you are open to these opportunities, you can stay receptive and proactive in pursuing your financial goals. These declarations then translate into concrete thoughts, thoughts become actions, and actions lead to results. While it may seem easy on paper, it can become complicated to actually implement and strategize your financial moves and goals.

By shifting your mindset, utilizing the power of compound interest, budgeting effectively, reverse engineering your goals, and making simple money declarations, you can take control of your financial future. However, navigating the complexities of finance can be challenging, which is why I recommend seeking the guidance of a seasoned CERTIFIED FINANCIAL PLANNER™ like myself. With the right mindset and tools at your disposal, you can achieve financial freedom and live the life you desire.

# 10

# Choosing the Who to Help with the How of Finances

I would guess that about 90 percent of my clients were already collaborating with financial professionals, be they advisors, CPAs, or family friends, before working with me. They sought out my team and me either because their current approach didn't sit well with them, or they were interested in a new perspective on potential gaps in their planning. I like to believe they crossed my doorway after their inner Boss amplified its voice, prompting them to explore alternative approaches.

My firm, Aurion Wealth, is committed to promoting financial literacy through various channels, including radio, social media, speaking events, and our two podcasts: "Kin & Capital" and "Shear Wealth." As a result, we've been fortunate to help numerous people with their financial futures. The majority of our clientele, however, come either from satisfied existing clients or are referred by our network of CPAs and attorneys with whom we collaborate daily to create holistic financial plans.

Despite these varied sources, I've noticed several recurring themes from new clients:

- Members of their existing financial team aren't effectively collaborating.
- They're seeking a trustworthy second opinion due to past negative experiences with advisors or market losses stemming from poor advice.
- Their business or personal wealth has grown, and they're questioning the adequacy of their current financial plan.

- Their tax professionals offer limited strategies for shelter, deferral, and growth.

- They feel uneasy about their current financial situation and doubt that their existing plan addresses all their priorities.

- They've stayed with advisors they don't trust out of fear or complacency until a crisis makes change imperative.

- Their current advisor is retiring, and they're not comfortable with the replacement.

I want to clarify that I don't believe all advisors outside of my team are lacking. I've encountered many competent professionals throughout my career. However, I've also met many who seem lost. One prevalent issue is that some advisors aren't living lifestyles remotely similar to those of their clients. It raises questions about the efficacy of their advice, especially in areas like tax strategy and advanced estate planning. Given the industry's mixed reputation, it's important to ask some basic questions when selecting a financial advisor to partner with.

- **"Are you a fiduciary?"**
  - Most advisors who work for a broker/dealer are not; however, their firms have large enough compliance divisions that try to keep them on "the right track." A true fiduciary will always be acting in your best interest and may contain industry marks such as CERTIFIED FINANCIAL PLANNER™ (CFP® ) or be registered as an Investment Advisor Representative (IAR).

- **"How long have you been an advisor, and may I have two referrals?"**
  - A good advisor will have a roster of clients willing to advocate for them and provide some great insight into their personal experiences.
- **"How much do you charge? Do the funds have expense ratios?"**
  - Fees are very important to consider because too many fees can erode your returns. I left a job working for a broker/dealer to go to an RIA once I realized the unbelievable amount of fees brokers/dealers charge to the advisors with the expectation that the fees will be passed through to clients.
- **"Who is the custodian?"**
  - Knowing where the assets are held (the custodian bank) is important too. A custodian is a financial institution that holds customers' securities for safekeeping to minimize the risk of their theft or loss. It's like a big safe. Some examples of custodians are big banks like JP Morgan, Bank of America, and Wells Fargo, as well as Schwab, LPL Financial, Goldman Sachs, Fidelity, E*TRADE, Bank of NY/Mellon/ Pershing, and so on. They hold securities and other assets in electronic or physical form, just as a bank does, but they don't lend on those assets whereas banks often do.

- Since custodians are responsible for the safety of assets and securities (that may be worth hundreds of millions or even billions of dollars), they tend to be large and reputable firms. A custodian is sometimes referred to as a "custodian bank." Custodians also send notices to customers when certain activities are conducted on their behalf or using their assets. For example, when I buy or sell stocks for a customer, that person gets a message about it. They also send reports about what assets the person has.

These are all important questions to ask before you sign on with a new financial professional. Otherwise, you may find yourself the victim of poor investment moves, bad decision-making, or outright corruption. Does the name Bernie Madoff ring a bell? He masterminded the most notorious Ponzi scheme in history, which came crashing down in 2008. As the famed Warren Buffett insightfully remarked, "You only find out who is swimming naked when the tide goes out."[21] In 2008, the financial tide receded, revealing Madoff's deceit. His scheme passed as genuine primarily because he had control over the custodial company, which enabled him to manipulate funds at will. With this unchecked power, Madoff not only diverted money for personal gain but also falsified financial statements. These deceptive practices allowed him to trick some of the wealthiest people on the planet.

Numerous shows and movies have been created about corruption within the financial industry. Some of the most popular ones include *The Big Short*, *The Wolf of Wall Street*, and "Billions." These all show that bad people and bad advice do not have geographical limitations.

While my firm may manage your accounts, we have no direct access to your money. And believe me, I want it that way as much as you do. I don't ever want there to be a misappropriation of funds or risk or any possibility that the fault could lie with myself or my team. With this approach, we are both content.

## STRATEGIES FOR SUCCESS

I'll never forget the day Noah and Ashley walked into my office, exuding the confidence typical of successful business owners. Together, they had transformed their small tech startup into a multimillion-dollar enterprise in less than three years! However, when it came to navigating the intricate maze of investments, Noah and Ashley confessed that they felt lost. Despite their roaring success in the business realm, the world of investing remained an enigma. Noah shared how he'd been approached by numerous hedge fund managers and financial "gurus," each claiming to have a strategy that was the "golden path" to exponential wealth. Ashley said the financial jargon they hurled their way left her more perplexed than convinced. "We run a successful business, but this? It feels like a different planet," they both admitted.

"Don't even get me started on taxes!" Noah exclaimed. This is a sentiment I've seen echoed by many high-net-worth business owners, individuals, and retirees. Immersed in their ventures, they often lack the time or the inclination to decode the intricate ballet of the financial markets or the tax code. They just want to be able to work with someone they can trust and feel confident in without the fear of an ulterior motive.

I commiserated with them before speaking directly. Without confusing industry terms or judgments, I shared what I firmly believe:

- **No one owns the market:** First and foremost, it's crucial to understand that no one has a monopoly on market knowledge. While some strategies can offer robust returns during specific periods, the financial world's inherent volatility means no single approach is infallible.

- **Know your money script:** Over my 20-year career, I've gone deep into money scripts—the subconscious beliefs individuals harbor about money. These scripts, often rooted in childhood experiences and family values, profoundly impact financial behaviors. Exploring this for yourself will unlock meaningful growth for your future.

- **Assemble your support team:** Every successful business relies on a network of professionals, especially during its early stages when you might be juggling multiple roles. Speed up your journey to scaling and growth by identifying the right experts to manage specific tasks.

Key professionals like a CERTIFIED FINANCIAL PLANNER™, such as myself, alongside a CPA and an attorney are essential allies in your business journey.

- **Stay in the market:** In my observation, panicked feelings, while a common reaction to market downturns, are seldom beneficial. In many instances, widespread panic has exacerbated market downturns. As the legendary Warren Buffett aptly put it, the primary risk "comes from not understanding what you're doing."[22] Therefore, for investors to navigate these treacherous waters, a well-defined, disciplined action plan is paramount.

- **Grasp tax implications:** Understand the difference between short-term and long-term gains, especially in ventures like day trading where the tax nuances can greatly influence net earnings. For instance, when a stock is purchased and sold within a single year, any gains accrued are taxed as ordinary income. In contrast, if you hold onto an investment for more than a year, it's taxed at the more favorable long-term capital gains rate. This distinction becomes especially significant for those with an annual income exceeding $400,000; they could face a difference in taxation of 37 percent versus just 20 percent.

- **Be skeptical of real-time trading claims:** Immediate access doesn't always translate to accuracy or timeliness. Discern between genuine insights and outdated data masked as real-time content. For instance, disclosures from highly affluent individuals regarding their stock purchases can have significant delays. Consequently, by the time an average investor acts on this information, they might be making a move 45 days after the initial purchase by the wealthy individual.

After I reviewed these principles and established a foundation with them, I was able to get more specific with Noah and Ashley about their needs. I started with a three-pronged approach:

- **Dollar-cost averaging:** Noah and Ashley were no strangers to consistent effort and its rewards in business. I introduced them to the dollar cost averaging strategy, which promotes regular investments over time, cushioning against the whims of market peaks and troughs. To get started, you can simply invest monthly in an index fund or ETF. They are diversified and low-cost; they are groups of stocks in a bundle.

- **Writing covered calls:** For someone like Noah, who was willing to leverage some of his holdings for additional returns without excessive risk, writing covered calls presented an excellent opportunity. It allowed him to earn premiums while still participating in potential upside, offering a balance between risk and reward.

- **Dividend-paying equities:** I steered Ashley, a slightly more conservative investor, toward blue-chip companies known for consistent dividend yields. These companies, with their proven track record, were akin to the stable business contracts she so valued in her enterprise.

Beyond just focusing on their investments, we took a holistic approach to financial planning, crafting a well-protected and well-planned path. They appreciated my straightforward approach that didn't necessitate deciphering complex jargon or chasing after the next big thing. After crafting a comprehensive financial roadmap for them, I introduced Noah and Ashley to a highly skilled CPA and an attorney. As a united team, we collaborated to devise and implement strategies that not only met their present needs but also safeguarded their future. Our collective efforts ensured they stayed on course, providing both stability and direction for their financial goals and business endeavors.

Building wealth through investing, much like cultivating a thriving business, is a journey. It doesn't hinge on one-off tactics or riding the latest trend. Instead, it rests on sound strategies that when implemented consistently, can pave the way to genuine financial prosperity. Noah and Ashley's journey reinforced the idea that while the market's vastness and complexity might seem daunting, armed with the right strategies, team, and guidance, anyone—whether a novice investor, retiree, or successful business owner—can navigate their way to financial success.

# THE PATH TO WEALTH

*Creating* wealth is more than a stroke of luck or a fortunate inheritance. As the owner of a wealth management firm for nearly two decades, I've discovered that *building* wealth is an intentional journey. While the allure of fast riches might tempt many, genuine prosperity often eludes those who don't equip themselves with the right knowledge. If you have ever found yourself confused about finance, tax, insurance, or investments, know that you are not alone, and there is no shame in that. However, this lack of knowledge can be a stumbling block. Your willingness to learn is a clear indication of your dedication and optimistic perspective on your future.

Most people are worried about "losing money" in the stock market without realizing that they could "run out of money" in retirement by not investing at all. Did you know that the average annualized return on the S&P 500 is 9.82 percent? That's since its inception in 1928 through December 31, 2022! The average annualized return since adopting 500 stocks into the index in 1957 through December 31, 2022, is 10.15 percent.[23] This suggests that the chance of prospering in the stock market is generally favorable, a fact not often highlighted in the news. For two decades, my journey in the investment sphere has been molded by a potent mix of curiosity, discipline, and unwavering adherence to my investment principles. It's fascinating how fears of low-probability events can dominate our thoughts, a phenomenon mirrored in our everyday worries and relationships. How often do we fret about scenarios without actually considering their likelihood of happening? And how frequently do we construct anxieties instead of challenging them with factual information? Don't let this become your financial reality!

The stock market powers global economies, yet it's a space where even those with PhDs, with law degrees, or born into wealth can make irrational decisions. Intelligence doesn't make someone immune to mistakes. The market is a world filled with knowns, unknowns, and unknown unknowns. Early in my career, I too was naïve and worried about losing money in the markets. My initial success led me to uncharted territories that clashed with my personality. However, with time, I learned to invest based on facts and to remove emotions from investing, adhering to tried and true processes that can reduce ego-driven mistakes. The 2008 market drop surprised many, but for me, it was a moment of clarity. Rather than panicking, I found myself consumed by a passion for understanding the markets. My fascination with the stock market machine grew from there, driven by a desire to help others and a never-ending hunger for knowledge.

Considering the inherent volatility influenced by external factors such as recessions, wars, elections, and pandemics, it is vital to remember that fluctuations in the market are a natural part of the process. If you're going to do investing on your own, then here is some essential advice: instead of treating investments like a game of chance, it's wiser to focus on long-term ownership, your alignment with a firm's vision, and an understanding of its core fundamentals. Essentially, you should have a compelling reason to buy the stock in the first place. Luck can sometimes be better than strategy, but choosing a winning stock with a 900-times multiple is about as probable as that winning lotto ticket. You can passively invest through index funds and a handful of blue chips, or you can hire a financial team to do your investing for around one percent a year. Even if you hire someone, strive for a comprehensive understanding of the figures presented to you so you gain the full picture. It's important to note that investing is just one piece of the puzzle in your financial journey. As you traverse these pages, you'll realize that harmonizing various elements is pivotal for overall success.

When I work with clients, my strategy is clear and straightforward: prioritize top-notch companies with outstanding products, solid financials, and consistent growth. By partnering with industry experts, I can focus on my strengths, like crafting detailed financial plans and assembling the best team for each client. Smart investing goes beyond just the numbers—it's about understanding our need for safety and consistency. Wealth opens doors to personal growth. You can even use it to make a positive difference in the world. Achieving financial success is about continuous learning, smart planning, and steady progress. By making wise choices and focusing on what truly matters, we not only improve our financial health but also contribute positively to the wider community.

# KNOW THE REAL WORTH—TAX INCLUDED!

I believe that one of the most commonly overlooked aspects of financial planning is understanding taxes. Taxes can have a significant impact on your financial future, yet many people don't understand how they work or how to plan for them. This is where I come in with proactive strategies to help my clients plan for taxes ahead of time rather than simply reacting to them after the fact like some CPAs. I've been polishing my skills for over two decades, learning about the gaps in various planning opportunities, and finding ways to fill them. Tax professionals usually have the right tools to help most clients, especially those with incomes of a million dollars or less. They help set up multiple entity planning, qualified plans, and more, enabling income shifting and optimizing expenses. However, when clients earn substantially more, the available strategies often fall short, and traditional saving methods don't make much impact due to income levels.

Proactively planning for taxes can help minimize tax liabilities and maximize overall financial success. This includes strategies like tax-advantaged accounts, charitable giving, estate planning, and understanding how to offset capital gains and losses. Remember the example earlier about Taylor's Pension Max Plan? That strategy will save her $1,200,000 over those 16 years of investing. By working with me, my clients have peace of mind knowing that their financial future is being thoughtfully planned and managed. Don't let pride or shame stop you from taking practical action. Finances can be very complicated, and no one expects you to know everything—that is why these professions exist! You can afford what you can. If you want more, then you have to figure out the skills, mindset, and tools you need and who you need to work with to achieve that lifestyle.

## Strategic Tax Reduction Strategies: The Three Steps to Leverage Positive Arbitrage

Navigating the complexities of the tax system can be a daunting task. However, with strategic planning, it's possible to significantly defer, reduce, and in some cases, eliminate your tax liabilities. Here is a potential three-step tax strategy if your income is moving into the highest tax bracket zone. Unless you inherit cash like on an episode of "Succession," your income is your greatest wealth-building tool. If you're able to sway from the temptations of giving your income to the wrong investments too early, like cars, watches, clothes, and other non-appreciating asset classes, then you may be able to hit your path to success faster. Once you do, taxes will become a central concern.

1. **Use assets with unrealized capital gains:** Consider using assets you own like stocks, businesses, or real estate that have appreciated in value but *haven't been sold*. These unrealized gains are not taxable—*yet*. For example, real estate can offer a quick win. Buy below market value, invest in improvements, and increase its worth without incurring immediate tax liability.

2. **Leverage positive arbitrage:** Secure a low-interest loan against your unrealized capital gains. The goal is to reinvest this loan in opportunities with higher returns, creating a beneficial spread between the loan interest and the investment yield (which is called positive arbitrage). Note: exercise caution. Ensure the spread is sufficient to offset potential risks. Loans themselves are not taxable, providing a lump sum free from taxation.

3. **Acquire depreciable assets:** Use the loan to purchase assets that can be depreciated, like investment property or businesses with heavy machinery. Even if the asset appreciates in value, you can still claim depreciation, which serves as a tax shield. This strategy can offset other income and reduce your overall tax liability.

The goal is not just tax reduction; it's achieving financial freedom. The essence of this freedom is encapsulated in seven simple words: "Cash flow exceeds daily wants and needs." So, take these strategies to heart, recognize your needs, and set out to find the right professionals to offer you the support you deserve. After all, finances aren't *that* scary.

# 11

# How to Keep It All Together

You've come a long way. From identifying obstacles to using the 7-28 Method, from learning to communicate better to managing your finances, you've covered a lot of ground. But the work isn't over. The challenge now is to keep the momentum going.

It's easy to slide back into old habits. A missed workout or a skipped budget review can quickly turn into a string of excuses. But these setbacks don't define you. For me to really change, it was about confronting the truth: I was operating in a culture of immediacy, and it was holding me back. A culture of immediacy means the fire alarm is always going off, and you're so caught up trying to address emergencies that you never get the chance to look at your goals. But even fire stations have an action plan and protocols in place.

For over a decade, I found myself caught up in drama from every social circle I was in. I was constantly juggling the demands of my work and the challenges in my relationships. But looking back, I realized that much of the drama was either invented or created by me. Instead of taking control of my situation, I was always putting out fires and jumping from one problem to the next. Things had to change. I learned that by taking responsibility for my actions and reactions, I could avoid getting sidetracked by unnecessary drama. I also realized that I had to prioritize my own well-being and mental health, and I began to make self-care a priority.

Over time, these habits helped me regain my sense of control and confidence. I was no longer constantly reacting to drama around me, but instead, I was able to approach situations with a sense of calm and clarity. And while drama still occasionally arises, I now have the tools to handle it in a healthy and productive way.

It's not a one-stop checkpoint—I have a whole system in place when it comes to the sphere of health and wellness:

- **My calendar:** I'll admit it; I need a thoroughly organized, color-coded agenda to keep my life and my priorities straight. I'm usually scheduled out four weeks in advance, so my calendar can get pretty intense. To manage it all, I use a financial-planning-specific CRM system called Redtail.

- **My trainer:** I don't particularly love the gym, but I know I need it. So, what do I do? I meet with a trainer two to three days a week first thing in the morning, usually around 7 a.m. This routine makes it a no-brainer for me to show up, even if I'm still half-asleep. And guess what? Sometimes, when I'm feeling like a superhero with extra energy, I throw in a second workout either at the crack of dawn or after a long day of work. But here's the best part: once I'm at the gym for my usual session, my trainer takes charge. They become the drill sergeant of positivity, constantly motivating me.

    A trainer might not be a perfect fit for everyone, but such is the reality of life—we each find different guides and mentors that align with us. I find a trainer helpful, and they assist me in gaining a deeper understanding of my health, my dietary patterns, and the implications on my well-being. It's all about being ahead of the game. By embracing personal accountability, we can deliver optimal outcomes. When on the move, I'm proactive about organizing my workouts and pinpointing suitable workout spots. While I've established various fitness spots at home or nearby, it's essential to recognize when a change is needed. Just as you might switch therapists or coaches, it's perfectly acceptable to transition to a different trainer. A new direction doesn't negate the value of the previous experience; it merely indicates evolving needs and preferences.

- **Myzone®:** My brother became a beacon of discipline and determination in early 2023, fully inspiring me. Despite his demanding life, he consistently prioritized fitness, shedding weight and gaining vitality. His dedication introduced me to a tool called Myzone®, which uses a wearable device to monitor your heart rate during exercise and measures workout intensity and caloric burn. This not only helped monitor my physical progress but also connected me to a supportive community. Having a structured fitness goal became vital as I embarked on my weight loss journey after my miscarriage. Paired with MyFitnessPal and Apple Health, I gained a comprehensive health and fitness overview that drove genuine dedication to achieve my goals.

- **MyFitnessPal:** While it may seem like a hassle, entering your dietary information each day is an important step in being accountable to your meal plan. I'll never forget the line, "You can't out-train a bad diet." It's so true! What you put in your body controls 85 percent of your results, and what you do for exercise is 15 percent of that outcome. It can be easy to let things slip or make excuses for unhealthy choices, but tracking what you eat helps you stay focused and aware of your habits. So, even though it may feel like a pain in the butt, it's a valuable tool in achieving your goals and living a healthier life.

- **My show pony self-care routine:** Let's dive into a sphere that sparkles, an arena that many find intriguing and yet elusive. Brace yourselves because now we're going to "talk glam!" That health and wellness sphere represents your self-care, whatever that may look like for you. I often find myself answering questions on this topic. Beauty upkeep is a domain that may not resonate with everyone but undoubtedly holds a special place for many women who relish maintaining their hair, skin, nails, and more. You see, it's not just about external presentation; it's also about reflecting success and control. I've always wanted to radiate that air of confidence, that immaculate presentation of a professional who's got everything under control: the "show pony."

Adopting the mantra, "Get up, dress up, show up," is more than just an attempt to look good. It's about inspiring yourself with positivity. An integral part of maintaining this outlook is a consistent self-care routine. For some, it may seem like an extra luxury, but for me, it's a cherished form of self-care. Now, this sphere is an endless topic with dozens of different things to discuss, but I'm going to share the routines and methods that have proven effective for me.

Every month, I put some life into my hair color with my sweet and sassy hair stylist, Rorie. This includes a fresh blowout a few times a month as well. Every three weeks, my nails and lashes receive their own TLC, and quarterly Botox and facial treatments keep my skin fresh and youthful. These regular self-care rituals have metamorphosed into therapeutic sessions where I rejuvenate myself. Over time, I've formed great relationships with these professionals, whom I consider close friends, making the experiences even more fulfilling.

In addition, my nightly skincare routine holds immense importance in my self-care regimen. No matter how exhausted or late it is, I never skip washing my face and removing all my makeup before retiring for the night. One of my first jobs was working at the beauty care counter for Lancôme during my freshman year of college. At that point, I had only a vague idea about the importance and complexity of skincare. During that time, my job required me to understand the skin layers and the impact of sun exposure. I cannot overstate the importance of protecting your skin from sun exposure, especially since I tragically lost a close friend to melanoma. Thus, it's vital to incorporate a daily moisturizer with SPF into your regimen and always ensure you're protected before stepping out into the sun. In addition, I ensure my body receives monthly massages to counter the muscle fatigue caused by consistent workouts, which helps alleviate lactic acid build-up and makes for a better recovery. My husband certainly aids in the "foot rubbies" department. Staying well-hydrated forms an integral part of my regimen as it's vital for overall health and lends a healthy glow to my skin. Adding to the mix, I fortify my diet with multivitamins like B-12 and biotin, amplifying my health and wellness further. You can get links to all these products and routines by visiting www.728method.com.

In essence, each aspect of this routine, although seemingly centered around physical aesthetics, is about self-nurturing. It's a way to honor yourself and invest time and effort into your well-being, serving as a daily reminder of your self-worth, just like the meticulous attention to detail required in building your net worth. Glam, after all, is not just an indulgence; it's a lifestyle!

Without these structures in place to keep me on track, I'm lost to the nebulous, and it's a miracle if I meet my goals. I'm not the type of person who leaves things to chance; that's why I put the work in to stay organized and define my goals. A lot of very fruitful things are a struggle. And you know, if greatness were easy to come by, then everybody would have it. That's why my trainer always says, "Greatness *isn't* for everyone." You can achieve your version of greatness by sticking to a schedule and staying accountable. So, what does your self-care routine look like? Is it meditating in the woods? Playing tennis with your kids? Luxuriating in a bath? All are good options to ground yourself and care for the vessel that carries you through every challenge to achieve your goals.

Studies have consistently shown that establishing a routine is a key factor in achieving success and maintaining a sense of stability in your life. In fact, a recent article in *Forbes* highlights the critical role of accountability in achieving one's goals, stating in its title: "Accountability and Success: You Can't Have One Without The Other."[24] And it's not just about feeling good—research has demonstrated that having a routine and being accountable can significantly improve mood, increase productivity, and even reduce stress levels.[25] These habits are essential for anyone striving to become a successful multi-faceted Boss because they provide the foundation for consistent progress and continued growth. By establishing and sticking to a routine, you can stay focused, motivated, and on track toward achieving your goals.

For me, that means I get up every morning and spend 30 to 45 minutes on my morning routine—make coffee, pet the dog, check the stocks, and do some self-awareness check-ins with myself through my board of directors. It's a grounding ritual of mine, and it works to cut the chaos out of my life and prepare me for the day. My husband and I are not always in the same place, but we still make a plan to talk every day on the phone or through FaceTime in order to include one another in our day. Consistency is key to accountability, so take the steps to make your goals a habit. Having a partner who shares these goals makes it a little easier. Hubby and I discuss our goals every morning for the day, and we are sure to check in at night to see how each of us did. We are each other's cheerleaders, always.

## OFF THE RAILS

It's important to remember that society's definition of success may not align with your personal goals and values. There are many external pressures that can influence how we perceive ourselves and what we hope to achieve, but ultimately, it's up to us to choose our paths. I fell into the trap of trying to live up to societal expectations and others' opinions, even when it meant sacrificing my desires and aspirations. I was so focused on making my side business successful that I didn't even realize it wasn't taking me in the direction I wanted to head. Looking back, I wish I would have just done better underwriting of the project from the get-go and not have blindly jumped in.

It's not easy to break free from external pressures and the influence of our egos. It can take a lot of self-reflection and hard work to put aside egos and prioritize our goals and aspirations. But it's important to remember that our egos are not the boss of us—we have the power to take control of our own lives and make decisions that align with our true desires and values. By recognizing our priorities and putting in the work to stay true to them, we can achieve success on our terms.

We can't always operate at 100 percent, but if a bad day is turning into a bad week and then a bad month, it's time to focus. If you get to the point where you're not in control, your next move should be calling up a trusted friend for that "Walk and B*tch" session, a therapist, or a life coach. Ignoring your problems will allow them to build until they're out of hand, and then you'll *really* struggle to get back on track. Sometimes, a whirlwind of emotions can lead people to make decisions they shouldn't—you need to break the pattern and find an external source for accountability.

As a headstrong Leo, I often find myself taking on more than I can handle. It's all too easy to become overcommitted and try to do everything at once, but I've learned that this approach can be counterproductive. Having it all doesn't mean *doing* it all! And having it "all" isn't always good. After all, who leaves an all-you-can-eat-buffet thinking, "Wow, that was a great idea! I moderated how much food I ate." Rarely anyone. The whole point of those places is to overeat for a cheap price. And while that's kind to our wallets, it's not as kind to our health. The same can apply to people who are perpetual over-committers. When I'm juggling too many tasks, it's difficult to give my full attention and energy to any of them.

Of course, it's not always easy to let go of the desire to do it all. I have a natural inclination toward taking charge and being in control. But I've learned that there's strength in recognizing my limitations and seeking support when I need it. By working with coaches in my spheres, I'm able to achieve greater success and fulfillment than I ever could on my own.

In business, sometimes we need an outside perspective to see things more clearly. This is why many companies bring in consultants—they can provide valuable insights and help us make better decisions. In my vast experience working with clients, I've observed that many people are hesitant to share their financial situations because they feel embarrassed or scared. They worry that by seeking help, they'll be giving up their power to make their own financial decisions.

But nothing could be further from the truth; whether it's a financial advisor, a consultant, a trainer, or a therapist, experts give you the support you need to make better decisions. They don't take the power away from you. By seeking help from experts, you actually become stronger for it. Acknowledge what you don't know, and be willing to get help to build your knowledge and understanding.

Therapy is not a one-time cure for everything. People think they can attend one session, and they're immediately going to be better. That's not how it works. A single therapy session won't fix things. As with everything else, you have to practice and regularly get involved in your therapy, healing, and growth.

Research shows that while people benefit from both long-term and short-term therapy, consistent meetings with a therapist can lead to more improvement.[26] Just like how you can't go to the gym one day and suddenly lose 20 pounds or build sufficient muscle, you need to be consistent, hold yourself accountable, and put in effort every single day to find your way out.

Therapy can be the key to unlocking deeper insights and understanding about ourselves. I struggled for five years before I finally sought help. Once I started therapy, however, I was able to uncover the root cause of my struggles, a combination of my ego and the people I surrounded myself with.

Without the help of my coaches or therapists, it's hard to say how long it would have taken me to come to this realization on my own. With their guidance and support, I was able to acknowledge the role that others were playing in my discomfort and start to make positive changes in my life.

People always wanted *something* from me, which, to me, felt like I had to constantly perform for them. But they also filled this need I had, even though it came at a high cost. I was treated like a show pony but was running through my life challenges like a racehorse; I was racing forward and taking on responsibilities and kept going and going—it was exhausting, and I was always on the verge of burnout. I realized that this behavior had to stop. I was a *workhorse*—grounded and steadily working toward my goals—not a show pony or a racehorse. It was a profound revelation for me, and in all likelihood, I may not have seen the racehorse role as a problem without outside help. I learned to check in with myself, which is a really hard thing to do, but I promise it can make all the difference. And getting help, that insightful support you need, can make this process a whole lot easier.

When I had that moment of clarity, I asked myself, *Am I reluctant to change? Am I being stubborn? Am I trusting others more than I'm trusting myself? Am I making somebody else the Boss of my life?* Those are the kinds of questions you need to ask yourself. Unknowingly, people often surround themselves with those who confirm their discomforts, and if that's the case, you'll never get the progress you're looking for in your life.

Once I recognized the pattern of allowing others to control my life, I started to embrace my solitude and surround myself only with people who would actually bring me happiness and calm and support my drive for growth. The list of people in my inner circle may be smaller, but the relationships are truer than ever before:

- My husband, who's my best friend and always willing to discuss ways to be healthy and improve ourselves;
- My right hand, Cathy, who has been with me for nearly 15 years now—she's family;

- My therapists, coaches, and trainers who push me to be better;
- My family and close friends who cherish me and provide unwavering support;
- The Confucious in my phone, Ramey, who gives me sage advice every time I need it; and,
- My career, which enables me to help and empower not only myself but thousands of others!

This is a true support network I've built over time that aids in my happiness, peace, ambition, work, and relationships. Most people possess a flawed understanding of their self-awareness, leading them to remain stuck in their *dis*comfort zones instead of exploring beyond their comfort zones. This causes them to become entrapped in an unending cycle of tolerating unjust demands imposed by others, which can adversely impact their mental well-being.

And here's the worst part: they're not even conscious of this cycle. To fix it, you need to know when people are taking advantage of you or when you're succumbing to a negative mindset. If someone is enabling your toxic behaviors, they're keeping you in a discomfort zone instead of giving you the kick you need to make positive changes. Therapy can really help you build your self-awareness. At least, it's helped me in every facet of my life.

## ONE SIZE DOES NOT FIT ALL

Through therapy, I embraced self-evolvement, realizing the need to seek help and challenge negative conditioning. Therapy provided a guiding light, emphasizing that forgiveness is about ourselves, not others. We can control our response to people's actions by managing our expectations and creating space for other emotions.

Achieving progress in therapy is similar to pursuing any other goal or skill, such as advancing in your career. It requires consistency and practice. Therefore, it is crucial to establish a consistent and ongoing relationship with a therapist to experience meaningful change.

However, not every therapist will be the right fit. Different practitioners have their own methods and motivations, ranging from quick diagnoses to financial incentives. Some therapists will tell you what's wrong with you, some will suggest what your problem is and not even evaluate you, and some will literally want you as a client only to increase their paycheck—it's nothing more than a business for them. It's essential to do your research, taking the time to find a professional whose guidance aligns with your needs and objectives. Don't rush into a commitment just because a particular therapist worked for someone else. Make sure you choose a therapist who is the right fit for you. Don't pick someone at random and walk into their office. You also have to select a therapist whose advice you feel you'd be willing to accept. Take your time to find someone you can develop a relationship with and go from there.

As I reflect on my journey, I hope that this book can serve as a survival guide for others facing their own struggles and emotional turmoil. My goal is to provide comfort and guidance to the readers who can relate to the emotions and experiences that I share within these pages. I want you to know that you are not alone and that with perseverance and a willingness to confront your fears, you too can emerge from your trials with newfound strength and resilience.

When I find myself becoming increasingly angry or frustrated or experiencing panic attacks, it's a sign that I need to reflect on and understand the emotions that are driving my behavior. This allows me to gain greater control over my internal thoughts and reactions, effectively placing my "board of directors" in check.

Ultimately, seeking help is vital, regardless of the form it takes. Staying stuck in a state of turmoil only perpetuates suffering. There's no shame in asking for help; in fact, it's crucial for progress. Take that first step, and know that someone is always there to support you, waiting on the other side of the door.

## A COMMITMENT TO YOUR CAUSE

It's easy to look at a list of strategies and promise to follow through. Doing the actual work takes a whole lot more commitment. Above all, you need to take action. Be wary of overworking and burning down your energy. Life-changing habits go hand-in-hand with taking care of your greatest asset: yourself. Create a self-care schedule, and make sure you divert energy into that sector of your life so that you *can* have the strength and energy to fulfill your other goals. Your health and well-being are the foundational pillars that keep you moving forward and conquering every day. By committing to this sphere, you set yourself up for greater success. If this isn't your forte, seek expert help from a trainer, nutritionist, therapist, or a combination of the three. Investing in your health and well-being is the smartest move you can make. So, what are you waiting for?

# 12

# The Power of Taking Action

Congratulations! You have made it to the final chapter of *Meet Your Boss*. Most people tend to skip over the conclusion, but I encourage you to stick around for a few pages longer—I saved a few gems to give you that final kick off the couch. By this point, you have learned valuable strategies to improve your life, relationships, and financial situation. But the key to success is taking action.

Grab a sheet of paper and draw a circle. Pretend that circle is a wheel. Your mindset, health, relationships, emotions, financials, environment, and spirituality are the spokes of the wheel. One can't be shorter than the other; the pieces need to be uniform and in balance if the wheel is to rotate every day without falling apart. Being self-aware helps you recognize which spoke is getting dulled down, which needs a little TLC, and how fast or slow your wheel is spinning. I'm a big believer that you can devote energy to all seven parts of your wheel—that's what it means to be well-rounded. And you need to keep your wheel well-oiled every single day.

The wheel spins fast if you're hungry. Hungry to achieve, grow, develop, and win. You need to be hungry for *more*. It is easy to read books and attend seminars, but it is much harder to act and implement the strategies you have learned. As you prepare to close this book, take off your rose-colored glasses, give yourself a good look, and see what's been holding you back. It's time to make some changes. Here are seven tips for taking action and making the most of the strategies you have learned in this book:

1. **Create a plan:** Develop a plan for implementing the strategies you have learned. Break the plan into smaller, achievable goals that you can work toward every day.

2. **Prioritize:** Determine which strategies are most important to you, and focus your energy on those first. Don't try to do everything at once or you'll burn out.

3. **Be consistent:** Consistency is key to achieving your goals. Make a commitment to yourself to work toward your goals every day, even if it is just a small step toward a larger goal.

4. **Celebrate small successes:** Celebrate every small success as it will keep you motivated and encouraged to keep going.

5. **Don't be afraid to ask for help:** Support from friends, family, or a professional can be invaluable in achieving your goals. Don't be afraid to ask for help when you need it.

6. **Embrace failure:** Failure is a part of life, and it is how we learn and grow. Don't be discouraged by setbacks. Instead, use them as opportunities to learn and improve.

7. **Stay positive:** A positive attitude is essential to success. Surround yourself with positive influences and stay focused on your goals.

Remember, taking action is the most critical step in achieving your goals and taking charge of your life, love, and financial future. Life is not a spectator sport; you must participate and play if you want to win. If you don't know how to do something right off the bat—your job, finances, even self-reflection—then roll your sleeves up and *learn*. I recall being halfway through a workout, feeling drained and overwhelmed. As I attempted to proceed, the weight seemed unbearable. That's when my trainer leaned in and said, "Amanda, it's not heavy; it's just hard." He was spot on. I realized I was fully capable of pushing through; I just had to give it my all. By applying this same idea of pushing through, learning something new, and participating at your maximum ability, progress becomes achievable. No one can carry you into this progress. It is up to you to use the strategies you have learned in this book, put them into action, and dedicate effort to growing each day. With hard work, commitment, and perseverance, you can create the life you want and deserve. Meeting your inner Boss and taking charge of your life is no easy feat, but it's time to accept that role.

*You are the Boss of your life. Nice to meet you.*

# ACKNOWLEDGMENTS

"Appreciation is a wonderful thing. It makes what is excellent in others belong to us as well"

— Voltaire[27]

Countless acquaintances, friends, family, and colleagues have intertwined their journeys with mine, entrusting me not only with their visionary ideas and personal narratives but also with their financial lives. This profound trust has allowed me to exceed my potential and realize the depth of my capability. Each story within this book is enriched by their valuable contributions, making every interaction a cornerstone and delight of my professional and personal journey. A special nod to my amazing husband, Andy, and my right hand, Cathy, who have been unwavering pillars of support, offering themselves for daily introspection and reflection. Their patience and understanding have been priceless. Moreover, my friends, my family, and even those whom I've met briefly have contributed significantly to my growth and understanding. Every encounter has been an opportunity to learn, reminding me that wisdom can come from the most unexpected places. Finally, my publisher's belief in the value of my story, coupled with their expert guidance, has helped transform this book from an idea into reality.

# BONUS STORIES

## WANT MORE TIPS AND ADVICE FROM THE BOSS HERSELF?

## FIVE PIECES OF PSYCHOLOGY WISDOM

Nobody wants their emotions to hijack them, a situation that is often rooted in a dysregulated nervous system. Though I don't possess a psychology degree, my thirst for knowledge has led me to devour countless books on health and lifestyle. I've also had the privilege to gain insights from physicians, therapists, and self-care "gurus," many of whom are my clients. My mission here isn't to prescribe medical advice but to share wisdom that might inspire others to take control, transforming their lives from the inside out.

1. **Unaddressed pain morphs:** Pain, when neglected, transforms into more insidious forms of suffering.

2. **Denial isn't a path to healing:** True resolution comes from confronting pain directly, not burying or ignoring it.

3. **Life scripts:** Every individual operates from a subconscious script that affects their thoughts, actions, and interactions.

4. **Values over pleasures:** Lasting contentment comes from upholding genuine values rather than chasing transient pleasures.

## ADDITIONAL FINANCE RESOURCES

Women tend to be more nurturing and risk-averse, and this attitude often stretches to their finances as well. In many modern-day households, women are the breadwinners, not the men. Husbands no longer need to be in control of their wives' purses. Women are becoming more and more empowered to take charge of their finances, and it's about time too. There's an endless supply of resources available to build your foundation of financial literacy.

My clients at Aurion have custom financial pages to track their progress, investments, and important documents. There are also plenty of other great financial resources like Mint, NerdWallet, BankRate, and Investopedia. Through these, you can create budgets, set up bill payments, or prepare for retirement or travel. And there are numerous blogs with tips for investing, mortgage refinancing, and insurance—there's even a section for business owners! Don't let your ego get in the way of making optimal financial choices.

Beyond these outside resources, I keep an updated resource center on my site, www.aurionwealthadvisors.com. Regardless of your needs and stage of life, I have videos and articles to answer some of your most pressing questions.

## BUDGETING: THE FOUNDATION OF FINANCIAL PLANNING

Budgeting is crucial to financial planning, yet it's often overlooked. I can't tell you how many people of all levels of wealth have zero idea of what they spend. According to a study by Debt.com, eight in 10 Americans budget their money, though this doesn't account for the number who successfully *follow* their budget.[28] That said, I highly encourage you not only to set a budget but to stick with it. A lack of budgeting leads to overspending and the inability to save for retirement. There are fundamental, basic rules of thumb to follow when budgeting. Twelve months is typical, but shorter time periods can be used if annual income and expenses cannot be estimated. Below are some guidelines for establishing a budget:

- Make it flexible;
- Make it simple;
- Estimate unknowns and different variables; and,
- Project expenses (typically projected out one year).

Adopting simple principles like the 50/30/20 rule (where half your income goes to necessities, a third to luxuries, and a fifth to savings) can pave the way to fiscal discipline. Additionally, fixed housing costs shouldn't surpass 28 percent of gross income, and total debt shouldn't exceed 36 percent. Exceed these, and you might be living unsustainably. In a higher interest rate environment, combined with inflation, I see that number dropping to even 20 percent for the fixed housing costs.

Financial literacy is a critical aspect of personal finance that impacts individuals and communities at large. Only 33 percent of adults worldwide are financially literate, meaning 3.5 billion adults globally lack an understanding of basic financial concepts, suggesting deep disparities in financial knowledge around the world. This highlights the need for more financial education and literacy programs to help people understand basic financial concepts, which can help them make better financial decisions and improve their overall financial well-being. If you're aware of a gap in your knowledge, don't be afraid to bring in an expert. Misinformation feeds the masses, especially because of social media. You can't rely on an Instagram post to educate you on what to do with your money or take advice from a Tweet on the security of your investment. If you realize that you're out of your depth when it comes to planning financially, you should defer to someone else. This brings to mind a relevant adage: "The market can remain irrational longer than you can remain solvent."

Our website (www.728method.com) offers a plethora of free E-books and educational resources covering a wide range of financial topics, including budgeting, investing, and debt management. Whether you're just starting your financial journey or looking to refine your existing knowledge, our resources are designed to provide you with the information and tools you need to succeed.

# THE ROMANTIC FINANCE TALK

I want to talk to the couples now. Don't wait for a major life event to have your first "money talk." Living together already entails financial adjustments. So, discuss your individual and shared financial expectations early on to avoid unpleasant surprises. Here are some guiding questions:

- Do your financial priorities align or complement each other?
- How much do you want to contribute to an emergency fund each month?
- What's the ratio between your joint income, spending, and saving?
- How often will you assess your financial standing?
- How separate or integrated do you want your finances to be?

These questions require careful thought and a shared commitment. It's essential for couples to communicate openly about income, debts, and differing money mindsets. If you're with the right partner, they should appreciate your proactive approach. This could even extend to considering a prenuptial agreement, which is more than just an "exit plan." It's a contract that can help you avoid complicated, costly, and emotionally draining divorces by setting clear financial terms.

## Take It Seriously

Tackling these questions is not a casual affair. It takes time, consideration, and commitment. Open communication is critical to ensure that these important financial discussions don't devolve into tension-filled, one-sided dialogues. Take it seriously—so seriously, in fact, that you might consider consulting financial and legal advisors before entering into marriage.

Proper financial planning can not only save money but also marriages. My firm frequently testifies in high-stakes divorce cases where previous poor financial planning led to years of legal battles and exorbitant fees. So, if you're contemplating marriage, especially as a high-net-worth individual, seek professional guidance. It's a responsible step to take for your financial future.

## Do You Have a Plan B?

Many people only consider Plan A and neglect to think about Plan B. With a strong money mindset, you'll embrace the realization that what you earn is yours to manage. Even in my relationships, I knew that if I were to end up alone, I'd still be financially secure because I'm in control of my financial future. Staying in jobs or relationships because of financial fears limits your growth and independence. That's why having a Plan B is essential regardless of whether you're married or single.

A Plan B might be a separate account that serves as a financial safety net in case you lose a job or experience a change in your relationship. It could mean titling your assets in a separate LLC or trust to protect against a business deal that goes sideways. Or maybe it's time to look at life insurance, which is a selfless act to ensure loose ends are covered if something were to happen to you.

While it might feel awkward initially, such preparation is actually a rational step to protect both yourself and your loved ones from unforeseen circumstances. A backup plan encourages conversations about financial security within your relationships.

## The Marriage Blueprint: Your Nuptial Operating Agreement

In my decades of working with business owners, not a single one has referred to their initial business plan as a "pre-biz plan." They call it an operating agreement. This agreement outlines the beginning, middle, and possible ends for the business—covering various scenarios like selling, dissolving, or even adding more partners. (You could do the same in your marriage if you're into that sort of thing.) So, forget about old-school prenuptial agreements that only focus on exits—I like to call this "the marriage blueprint." Consider the marriage blueprint a comprehensive guide for navigating the financial intricacies of your partnership. Here are the seven key topics your blueprint should cover:

- **Financial Foundations:**
  - **Assets and liabilities:** Take inventory to ensure transparency and avoid surprises.
  - **Income and expenditures:** Establish a joint or proportional system for daily expenses and discuss your various income streams.
- **Investment Strategy:**
  - **Future goals:** Outline mutual financial objectives, such as buying a home.

- **Investments:** Agree on a joint investment strategy and where these funds will be kept and managed.

- **Family and Life Planning:**
  - **Family planning:** Discuss financial provisions for potential children, including education and welfare.
  - **Long-term care:** Decide what resources will be used and the preferences for long-term care if one of you becomes ill.

- **Retirement Readiness:**
  - **Retirement accounts:** Agree on retirement account types and the amount each will contribute.

- **Emergency Preparedness:**
  - **Emergency funds:** Create a fund for unexpected life events.
  - **Inheritance and gifts:** Outline how you will handle gifts and inheritance received during the marriage.

- **Property and Possessions:**
  - **Real estate:** Discuss existing properties, whether to sell them or buy new ones together.
  - **Business ownership:** Decide whether and how each partner has a stake in the other's business.

- **Flexibility and Contingencies:**
  - **Amendments:** Make it amenable to reflect lifestyle and goal changes.

- **What-if scenarios:** Include provisions for changing circumstances and possible exit strategies.
- **Insurance:** Is the family well-protected if something happens? Are the "what if" plans funded adequately, and from where?

Your marriage blueprint should be a comprehensive guide for both partners. It's not just a document; it's a dynamic roadmap that adapts as your relationship evolves. Marriages are rarely perfectly 50–50 because everyone's situations are different. Focus on what works for you and your spouse. With all the *T*s crossed and the *I*s dotted, this blueprint can be your go-to manual for a financially harmonious life together.

## Balancing Power Couples: A Tale of Equal Success

High-profile, equally-successful couples face unique challenges when it comes to managing finances. My firm specializes in helping such couples explore creative financial strategies to ensure mutual benefit during the marriage while also offering protection should the marriage not work out.

For instance, Alex and Jordan, both of whom are successful in the tech industry, opted for a joint investment account alongside their separate business funds. Taylor and Casey, renowned musicians, created a family trust to manage their combined wealth.

When it comes to real estate, the decision to sell or keep properties is also significant. We help couples analyze current market values, tax implications, and long-term goals to make informed choices that align with their marriage blueprint.

## Picking Up the Pieces: Financial Planning After Divorce

Transitioning from the marriage blueprint to a new financial chapter post-divorce may be challenging, but it's not insurmountable. Emotional upheavals are a given, but you'll find stability in numbers. Here's how to find your financial footing when facing divorce:

- **Schedule a money date:**
  - Dedicate two hours solely to go through your financial situation in detail.
  - Whether it's a cozy cafe or your living room, choose a space where you can focus. Equip yourself with a laptop, calculator, calendar, and all your account passwords. This proactive step can alleviate some of the stress surrounding financial uncertainty.

- **Define your goals:**
  - **Short-term goals:** Outline your immediate needs for the next year, whether it's new furniture or a restorative vacation. Get as specific as possible and assign approximate costs to each.
  - **Long-term goals:** Reflect on long-term objectives like retirement planning, funding children's education, or moving to a new city. List these along with any questions you might have to discuss with an advisor.

- **Calculate your income:**
  - Document every source of income, including your monthly paychecks after taxes, alimony, child support, and other passive incomes.
  - Sum it up to arrive at your total monthly income. This is the financial resource pool you'll be working with.
- **Itemize expenses:**
  - **Fixed expenses:** Catalog your mandatory monthly payments like rent, utilities, and groceries.
  - **Variable expenses:** List optional expenditures like shopping, dining out, and leisure activities. Include a category for "fun money" as emotional well-being is crucial during these times.
- **Balance your budget:**
  - Compare your income to your expenses to see how much wiggle room you have. If the numbers don't add up, you may need to adjust. Start by revisiting variable expenses and identify areas to cut back. Then, think of ways you could increase your income.
- **Assemble your team:**
  - Your team should include professionals like a CERTIFIED FINANCIAL PLANNER™, divorce lawyer, and accountant. Adding friends, therapists, or a life coach can offer emotional support and additional accountability.

- **Implement and monitor your plan:**
  - Utilize budgeting software to keep track of your finances. At our firm, clients can sign up for their own comprehensive "My Aurion Plan," a personal financial planning portal at www.aurionwealthadvisors.com to assist them in staying on course.
  - Regularly consult your support team, and update them on your financial progress, making adjustments to your plan as necessary.

By carefully implementing these steps, you're setting the stage for a financially stable future. You also will have your marriage blueprint ready to go if you want to get married again! Change may be daunting, but remember, you have the resources and resilience to come out stronger and more financially secure.

## THE NEXT GENERATION: RETHINKING HOW WE TEACH KIDS ABOUT MONEY

After establishing or even re-establishing your financial footing—be it post-divorce or simply revisiting the marriage blueprint—it's essential to consider how you'll pass on financial wisdom to the next generation. Our early experiences often set the stage for our adult attitudes toward money, and my journey is a testament to that.

Growing up, the emotional distance I felt from my parents inadvertently distorted my perception of money. It was either a punitive measure or a manipulative tool rather than a resource to be wisely managed. This absence of positive reinforcement took a toll on my self-esteem and led me to internalize a mindset of scarcity and financial fear.

This realization sparked a curiosity in me to explore better methods of imparting financial literacy to children—methods that empower rather than instill fear. Before we go into those alternative teaching techniques, it's important to recognize and unpack some of the traditional approaches that may have perpetuated unhealthy financial attitudes for many of us.

- **Allowance for chores:** Parents often pay their kids an allowance in exchange for doing chores around the house, teaching them that money is earned through work. The idea that money is only earned through hard labor and one must always work for it can instill a "workaholic" script. People may grow up thinking they constantly have to be working to deserve money, such as with the Money Vigilance script.

- **Saving in a piggy bank:** Many parents encourage their children to save money by putting it in a piggy bank, emphasizing the importance of saving which can foster Money Balance. However, this method could also lead to money hoarding, such as the Money Vigilance script, when it is overemphasized to a point where the kid develops anxiety about spending money and prefers to save it for undefined future needs, sometimes to the point of detriment to their current well-being.

- **Lecturing about frugality:** Parents sometimes lecture kids about the value of money and the importance of being frugal, often using phrases like "money doesn't grow on trees." Such teachings often lead to a scarcity mindset and a Money Avoidance script. Here, people may grow up to view money as a limited resource that might run out at any moment, which can lead to financial anxiety and an overemphasis on cost-cutting instead of value creation.

- **Budget lessons:** Some parents involve their kids in household budgeting activities like grocery shopping to teach them about the cost of living and budget constraints. These can result in a Money Vigilance script, prompting people to become overly cautious with their finances, continually concerned about making ends meet or achieving financial goals. While vigilance isn't bad, this can lead to financial stress and missed investment opportunities.

- **Fear-based warnings:** Parents often use cautionary tales or warnings about the consequences of poor money management, such as going into debt or not being able to afford necessities. Constant warnings about debt and financial ruin can instill a Money Avoidance script, where individuals develop a fear of managing their finances. They may think that wealth is bad and may subconsciously sabotage their financial success to avoid perceived negative consequences.

Here are the top seven classic sayings parents often use to teach kids about money. I also explore why they're flawed and should, perhaps, be retired from our societal teachings.

1. **"Money doesn't grow on trees."**
   - *Related money script: Money Avoidance*
   - This phrase often fosters a scarcity mindset, potentially leading to Money Avoidance, where people feel overwhelmed and fearful of managing their finances.

2. **"We can't afford that."**
   - *Related money script: Money Vigilance*
   - The frequent use of this statement reinforces a notion of scarcity and potential financial instability, leading to extreme caution and vigilance around money.

3. **"Rich people are greedy/evil."**
   - *Related money script: Money Worship*
   - This saying creates an unhealthy association between wealth and moral or ethical deficiencies, contributing to a Money Worship mindset where accumulating wealth is seen as a solution to all problems.

4. **"You have to work hard to earn a penny."**
   - *Related money script: Money Status*
   - This phrase may instill the idea that financial worth equates to personal worth, potentially causing a focus on Money Status through the acquisition of wealth or material possessions.

5. **"Don't talk about money; it's rude."**
   - *Related money script: Money Dependency*
   - By making money a taboo subject, this phrase may discourage financial literacy and independence, leading to a Money Dependency mindset where financial responsibility is outsourced to others.

6. **"It's just money; it's not important."**
   - *Related money script: Money Empowerment*
   - Contrary to the Money Empowerment script, dismissing money's importance can result in neglecting the potential of money as a tool for personal growth and positive impact.

7. **"You're just not good with money."**
   - *Related money script: Money Balance*
   - This phrase can negatively impact a person's ability to find a balanced approach to finances as it discourages the self-confidence required to maintain a Money Balance that values financial stability without overshadowing other life aspects.

Each of these classic sayings can play a role in shaping unhealthy money scripts, which can, in turn, influence your attitudes and behaviors toward finances throughout your life. Here are five new and improved methods to teach kids about money that align with healthy money scripts:

1. **Interactive budgeting games**
   - *Healthy money script: Money Empowerment and Money Balance*
   - **Why it works:** Make budgeting fun and interactive by using board games or apps designed to teach financial literacy. This approach encourages kids to view money as a tool for empowerment, giving them a balanced understanding of financial planning.

2. **Family investment discussions**
   - *Healthy money script: Money Empowerment*
   - **Why it works:** Include your children in simple conversations about investments and how they work. This provides an understanding of how money can grow and be used for future needs, fostering a sense of empowerment.

3. **Allocated spending jars**
   - *Healthy money script: Money Balance*
   - **Why it works:** Teach your child to divide their allowance or gift money into jars labeled "saving," "spending," and "giving." This holistic approach encourages balanced financial behavior, integrating saving, spending, and philanthropy.

4. **Role reversal shopping**
   - *Healthy money script: Money Vigilance and Money Balance*

- **Why it works:** Let your child take the lead in shopping for small items while on a budget. This exercise helps them become vigilant about spending choices and also allows for a balanced approach as they learn to prioritize needs over wants.

5. **Emotional spending conversations**

   - *Healthy money script: Money Avoidance (in a positive way by countering it)*
   - **Why it works:** Discuss the emotions that come with spending and saving. Make sure to correct any misconceptions and encourage an open conversation about financial anxieties. This can help prevent the development of a Money Avoidance script.

By adopting these improved methods, you can help your child develop a healthier, more constructive relationship with money, setting them up for financial wellness in adulthood. In addition, here are seven positive things parents can say to their children about money, aligned with the healthy money scripts you've outlined:

1. **"Let's plan how to spend your allowance together."**
   - *Related money script: Money Avoidance*
   - This encourages kids to confront financial decisions head-on rather than avoiding them by breaking down complex tasks into manageable ones.

2. **"Money is a tool; it's not good or bad by itself. It's how you use it that counts."**
   - *Related money script: Money Worship*
   - By portraying money as neutral, parents can teach their children to find joy in non-material things and not see money as the end-all-be-all.

3. **"It's okay to spend on things that are important to you, but let's also save for the future."**
   - *Related money script: Money Vigilance*
   - Encouraging a balanced approach to spending and saving can help kids become vigilant without becoming overly cautious or fearful.

4. **"Your value is not determined by how much money you have."**
   - *Related money script: Money Status*
   - This reinforces the idea that self-worth is separate from financial status, helping to build real connections and live authentically.

5. **"Let's talk openly about money. There's nothing to be ashamed of."**
   - *Related money script: Money Dependency*
   - Open discussions about money can foster financial independence and literacy, countering the mindset of financial dependency.

6. **"How can we use money to help others or make a positive impact?"**
   - *Related money script: Money Empowerment*

- This instills the value of using money for good, teaching kids that money can be a tool for personal growth and societal impact.

7. **"Money is part of life, but it's not everything. Let's focus on what truly matters."**
   - *Related money script: Money Balance*
   - This encourages a balanced view of money and its place in a well-rounded life, enabling a focus on overall well-being.

By using these positive sayings, parents can help their children form healthy money scripts that promote balanced and empowered financial behavior.

# HEALTH AND WEALTH: A PHYSICIAN'S PERSPECTIVE

*provided by Dr. Kevin Hoffarth MD, IFMCP*

Having worked with thousands of patients, I've gained fascinating insight into human nature: most of my female patients usually scour all corners of the internet for health advice and my male patients receive direction directly from their spouses. Only after exhausting these sources would either of them come to me. This begs the question of *why* we do this. Why do we leave so much on the table with matters as important as health?

Little did I know, I had spent decades doing the same thing with my financials. I sought advice from my dad, a physician, and my friends who seemed to be more money-smart than I was—that is, until they admitted to getting advice from *their* friends. And no one in this interconnected web was an actual financial advisor. Yet, for some reason, I chose not to seek out professionals who could understand my circumstances and lay out a personalized, well-defined plan for me.

When I was in my 30s—finally making money for the first time in my life after 12 years of post-secondary education—I was influenced by several acquaintances who were boasting about their substantial profits from buying and flipping homes. It was appealing. This "easy money" triggered a surge of dopamine in my brain, leading me to believe, in body and mind, that I could replicate their success. This activated my parasympathetic nervous system, which is linked to feelings of peace, bliss, and inner contentment. Consequently, my perception of quick and easy wealth was converted to a tangible powerful feeling that I knew all the answers to my financial future. Embarrassingly, it was all rooted in an uneducated and simplistic assumption.

Unaware of the full implications, I found myself with four properties in my portfolio at the worst possible time in the real estate market—2007. My stress escalated, my business partner turned out to be a crook, and eventually, I was forced to sell three of the properties just to remain solvent. It was a total bust. This nerve-racking period significantly impacted my health, prompting me to stop, reflect, and have a serious conversation with myself—or, as Amanda calls it, my internal board of directors—regarding my financial future. It was a sobering experience, to say the least.

It took years of dabbling in the stock market, making some and losing some, before I reached this point of clarity. I would often make more money year after year but never truly expand my financial literacy beyond basic investment ideas. It was got so bad it felt like my investments were making more money for the IRS through taxes than they were for me! I was getting tired of the soul-sucking and never-ending heavy tax burdens. I realized I needed to strategically change my way of thinking. I finally decided to seek the same quality guidance that I would often suggest to my patients. I needed an expert who was seasoned, someone who understood the domino effect of the micro-decisions I had been making up until now and could help me transform them into great opportunities. I needed to ditch all the generic cookie-cutter and Band-Aid advice and find the right person to steer my ship into a healthier territory.

I started with my built-in resource of recommendations: my patients. Every day at my practice, I am privileged to work with C-Suite people who run large companies and often partner with financial experts—for their business or otherwise. Why had I not thought to just ask them before? As humans, we tend to make decisions based on our emotions. We ask those whom we trust for advice and grudgingly expand this circle beyond our friends and family. Yet, these people, however well-meaning, know your situation only peripherally—it's like asking "Dr. Google" to pinpoint the source of your headaches and being told it's either allergies or a brain tumor. A headache could indicate either option, but Google is using a narrow understanding of your symptoms to "diagnose" you. Facts are only as valuable as the person who can also decipher it and prescribe a personalized solution. The same can be true of your financial health.

Enter Amanda Hayes-Blocksom, author of *Meet Your Boss*.

Amanda instantly met the criteria of a true professional. She started off by reminding me that it's not how much money you make but how much you *keep* that matters. Like any good quarterback, she immediately brought game-changing knowledge and strengths to my financial strategy. My experiences with a financial expert had involved me being sold to, whether it was in the form of a retirement plan or some life insurance. But Amanda was different. She had no interest in selling me anything. For her, the focus was rebuilding my foundation and planning the next steps from there. It was clear early on that she possessed the key ingredients I was seeking in a true professional. Amanda clearly saw the winning end game.

When I heard she was writing a book, I was thrilled. And sure enough, her book contains all the insightful how-to and expert advice on all facets of life. It is a must-read for anyone. Amanda addresses themes of how we make unconscious decisions that impact our wealth, and her guidance emphasizes informed financial decisions—it's this same wisdom that has reshaped my business' financial future, my family's future wealth, and, most importantly, relieved me of the deep financial uncertainty I'd carried for decades before meeting her.

My final advice is that you should always consider the quality of the advice you take, whether it's for medical or financial reasons. These spheres are finely interwoven into your overall quality of life, so the stakes are high. If I advise my patients how to get out of their own way in order to thrive, a financial professional should most certainly do the same for the health of your finances. Amanda fundamentally embraces this same philosophy in how she guides clients to ultimately reach financial freedom. Amanda's work is an essential resource for anyone seeking a balanced and healthy life, and let's not forget, eventual financial freedom.

Dr. Kevin Hoffarth MD, IFMCP
Owner of BioFIT Medicine, Austin, TX
Author of *Functional Medicine: The New Standard*

# NOTES

1.  "How to Use the Law of Attraction to Build the Life of Your Dreams," Tony Robbins, accessed November 17, 2023, https://www.tonyrobbins.com/business/law-of-attraction/.

2.  Noah Brandt, "Women in Business Statistics in 2023 (Latest U.S. Data)," April 2, 2023, https://ecommercetips.org/women-in-business/.

3.  "Warren Buffett's Words of Wisdom," *Forbes*, January 10, 2007, https://www.forbes.com/2007/01/10/leadership-managing-money-lead-manage-cx_hc_0110buffett_slide.html?sh=a04db082e0de.

4.  "Don't Be Afraid of the Solitude that Comes with Raising Your Standards," Epic Quotes, January 29, 2021, https://www.epicquotes.com/dont-be-afraid-of-the-solitude-that-comes-with-raising-your-standards-ebonee-davis/.

5.  Thomas A. Harris, *I'm OK – You're OK* (New York: Harper Perennial, 2004).

6.  "How Box Breathing Can Help You Destress," *Health Essentials*, August 17, 2021, https://health.clevelandclinic.org/box-breathing-benefits/.

7.   Dan Sullivan, *Who Not How: The Formula to Achieve Bigger Goals Through Accelerating Teamwork* (New York: Hay House Business, 2020).

8.   Steve Bates, "Forced Ranking" *HBR Magazine*, June 1, 2003, https://www.shrm.org/hr-today/news/hr-magazine/pages/.

9.   Michael T. Deane, "Top 6 Reasons New Businesses Fail," December 30, 2022, https://www.investopedia.com/financial-edge/1010/top-6-reasons-new-businesses-fail.aspx.

10.   Grant Cardone, *The 10X Rule: The Only Difference Between Success and Failure* (Hoboken, New Jersey: Wiley, 2011).

11.   Dale Carnegie, *How to Win Friends & Influence People* (New York: Gallery Books, 1998).

12.   Gary Vaynerchuk, "Podcast - Gary Vaynerchuk," accessed November 2, 2023, https://garyvaynerchuk.com/podcast/.

13.   Les McKeown, *Predictable Success: Getting Your Organization on the Growth Track—and Keeping It There* (Austin, Texas: River Grove Books, 2014).

14.   Noel Sales Barcelona, "Sufi teacher, philosopher, and poet Rumi said, 'The wound is the place where the Light enters you,'" *Medium*, October 24, 2017, https://noelbarcelona1980.medium.com/sufi-teacher-philosopher-and-poet-rumi-said-the-wound-is-the-place-where-the-light-enters-you-c13e6e22074a.

15. "Mark Twain Quotes," Brainy Quotes, accessed October 17, 2023, https://www.brainyquote.com/quotes/mark_twain_103535.

16. "Panic Disorder," National Institute of Mental Health, accessed October 13, 2023, https://www.nimh.nih.gov/health/statistics/panic-disorder.

17. "EMDR Therapy," Cleveland Clinic, March 29, 2022, https://my.clevelandclinic.org/health/treatments/22641-emdr-therapy.

18. Leo Newhouse, "Is Crying Good for You?" March 1, 2021, https://www.health.harvard.edu/blog/.

19. Carlie Porterfield, "U.S. National Debt Eclipses $31 Trillion for First Time," *Forbes,* October 4, 2022, https://www.forbes.com/sites/carlieporterfield/2022/10/04/us-national-debt-eclipses-31-trillion-for-first-time/.

20. "Research Statistic on Financial Windfalls and Bankruptcy," National Endowment for Financial Education, January 12, 2018, https://www.nefe.org/news/2018/01/research-statistic-on-financial-windfalls-and-bankruptcy.aspx.

21. "Swimming Naked When the Tide Goes Out," Money, April 2, 2009, https://money.com/swimming-naked-when-the-tide-goes-out/.

22. Benjamin Snyder, "7 insights from legendary investor Warren Buffett," May 1, 2017, https://www.cnbc.com/2017/05/01/7-insights-from-legendary-investor-warren-buffett.html.

23. J.B. Maverick, "S&P 500 Average Return," May 24, 2023, https://www.investopedia.com/ ask/answers/042415/what-average-annual- return-sp-500.asp.

24. Marguerite LeBlanc, "Accountability and Succes: You Can't Have One Without The Other," *Forbes*, September 8, 2020, https://www.forbes. com/sites/forbescoachescouncil/2020/09/08/ accountability-and-success-you-cant-have-one- without-the-other/.

25. Mariana Plata, "The Power of Routines in Your Mental Health," *Psychology Today*, October 4, 2018, https://www.psychologytoday.com/ us/blog/the-gen-y-psy/201810/the-power-of- routines-in-your-mental-health.

26. "Why is consistency important for therapy?" Evolve Therapy, October 2, 2022, https://www. evolvetherapymn.com/post/why-is-consistency- important-for-therapy.

27. "Quote by Voltaire," Goodreads, accessed October 13, 2023, https://www.goodreads.com/ quotes/113418-appreciation-is-a-wonderful- thing-it-makes-what-is-excellent.

28. Karen Bennett, "The average American household budget," September 26, 2023, https:// www.bankrate.com/banking/savings/average- household-budget/.

investment results or function as a predictor of how your investment will perform. It is simply an approximation of the impact a targeted rate of return would have. Investments are subject to fluctuating returns, and there can never be a guarantee that any investment will double in value.

# ABOUT THE AUTHOR

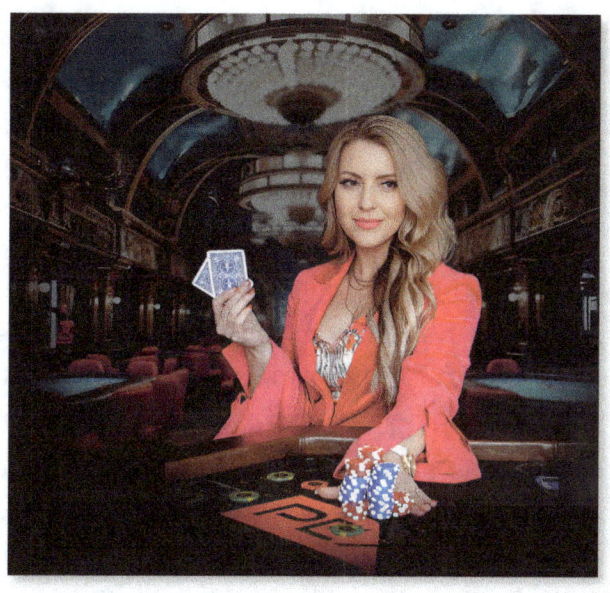

Amanda Hayes-Blocksom is a CERTIFIED FINANCIAL PLANNER™, the founder of Aurion Wealth and Aurion Wealth Advisors. Built on her passion for financial literacy and over two decades of industry experience, her firm caters to a diverse clientele. Amanda empowers her clients through her dedicated enthusiasm, meticulous care, and data-backed insights. To enhance her clients' financial journeys and life goals, she provides more than just advice; she offers a partnership for success.

Amanda is a steadfast advocate for financial education across all ages and is recognized through numerous industry honors. Frequently featured on radio, podcasts, and media outlets for her market insights, Amanda serves a diverse clientele, ranging from successful entrepreneurs to seasoned retirees and professionals. Her mission is to shoulder the burden of financial decision-making of clients who aspire to focus on their personal and professional ambitions, ensuring their financial trajectory aligns with their life goals.

Amanda's business ethos is rooted in the fusion of fervor and diligent consistency. This philosophy is mirrored in her personal pursuits, which include outdoor adventures like skiing and fishing, alongside a commitment to health and wellness. Quality time with her husband and family remains her most treasured activity, reinforcing her belief in a well-rounded existence.

Amanda's life strategy is encapsulated in the 7-28 Method, a comprehensive guide that harmonizes the essential facets of life from mental and physical health to financial stability and emotional well-being.